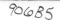

Image-Makers: Professional Styling, Hair and Make-Up

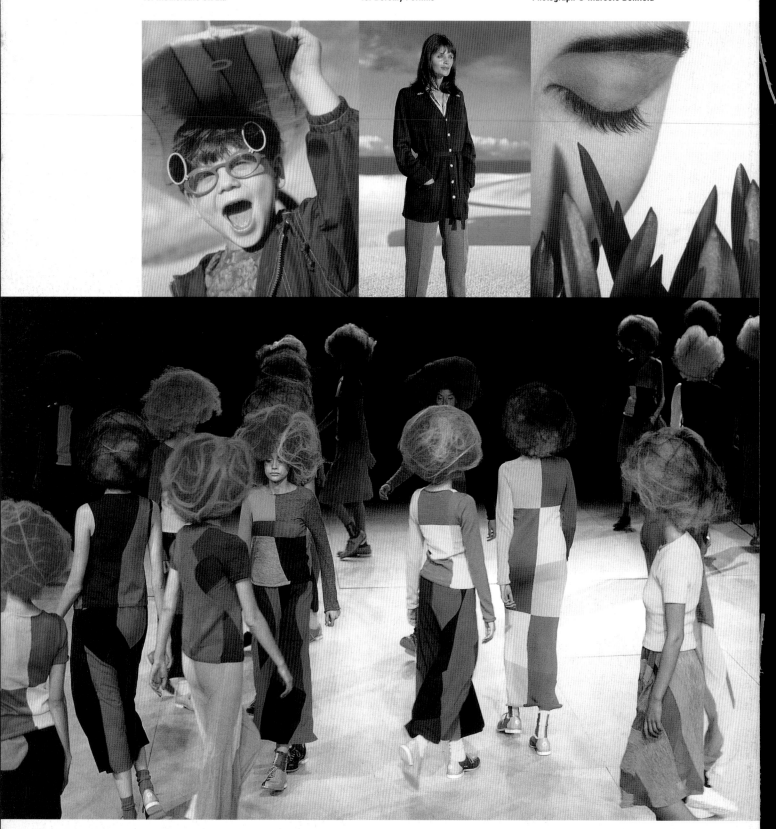

Photographer: Stefano Azario
for Mothercare UK Ltd

Photographer: Neil Kirk
for Dorothy Perkins

Photograph © Marcelo Benfield

Comme des Garçons
Photograph © Niall McInerney

Image-Makers: Professional Styling, Hair and Make-Up

Lee Widdows & Jo McGuinness

B T Batsford Ltd, London

© Lee Widdows and Jo McGuinness 1997
Photographs © as marked

First published 1997

Printed in Hong Kong
for the publishers
B T Batsford Ltd
583 Fulham Road
London SW6 5BY

ISBN 0 7134 7701 6

A CIP catalogue record for this book is available from
the British Library.

This book is dedicated to family and friends.

**The authors would like to thank the following for their
invaluable help in compiling this book:**

Stefano Azario, Davies Baron, Stephanie Churchill PR/
Dorothy Perkins, Sally Courtis, Helen Crowther, Rachel
Collingwood, French Connection, Heddi Greenwood, Sandro
Hyams, *Mail on Sunday*, Niall McInerney, Modus Publicity,
Mothercare UK Ltd, Next, Andy Robson, Tracey Sayer,
Julian Seaman, Anna Solowij, *Vogue*, Joy Wilson,
Ayshe Yusuf.

Contents

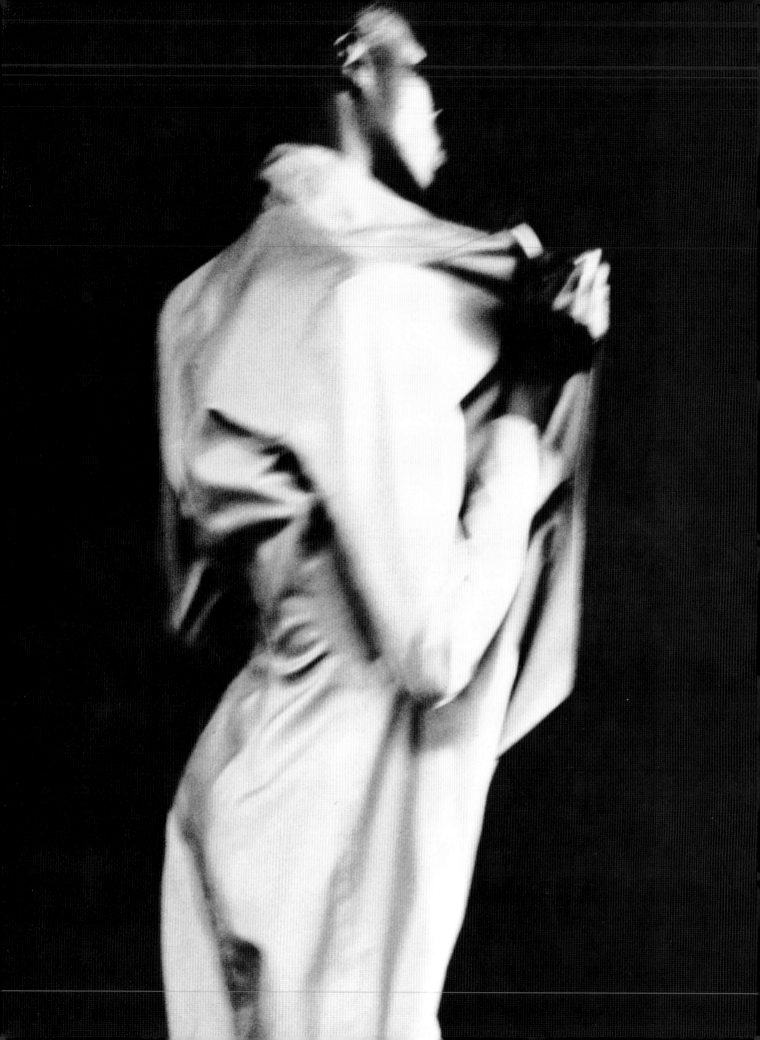

Introduction

Image-making is an integral part of our highly visual popular culture. Over the past decade, fashion image-making has become more rapid and disposable. New images have a short shelf life: they inspire and excite us, become dated and are left behind as quickly as fashion changes.

The image-making industry is about team work and the dynamics of a good creative team are essential. Working alongside the photographer, the stylist, hair stylist and make-up artist are the key players in the creation of a fashion image. These image-makers absorb changing ideas and cultural trends and reinterpret them as fashion, enjoying exciting and challenging careers.

Image-Makers examines the team responsible for the creation of fashion images. It introduces the different areas of styling and hair and make-up direction that relate to fashion, explaining what goes into the creation of a fashion image, be it for the runway, editorial fashion pages, advertising, catalogues or music promos.

The image-makers

Over the past 15 years, styling has become recognized as a respected profession. The influence of the stylist is not limited to fashion: celebrities, the music industry and even political parties turn to successful stylists for a new look.

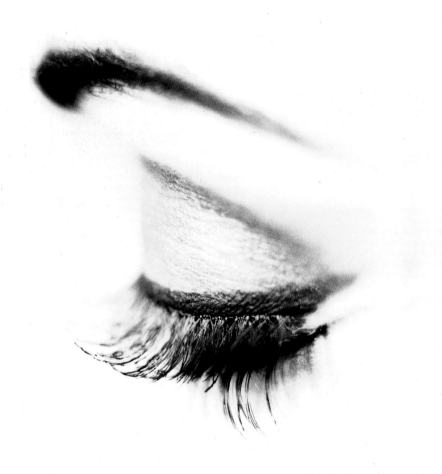

Photograph © Sandro Hyams
(left)

Issey Miyake
Photograph © Niall McInerney
(right)

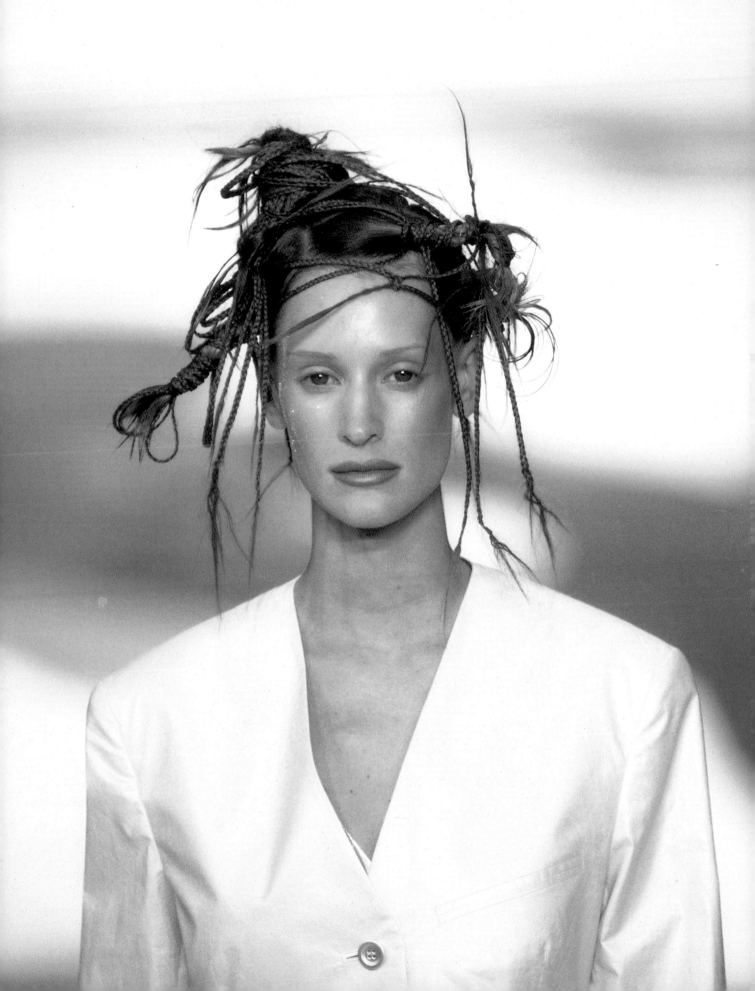

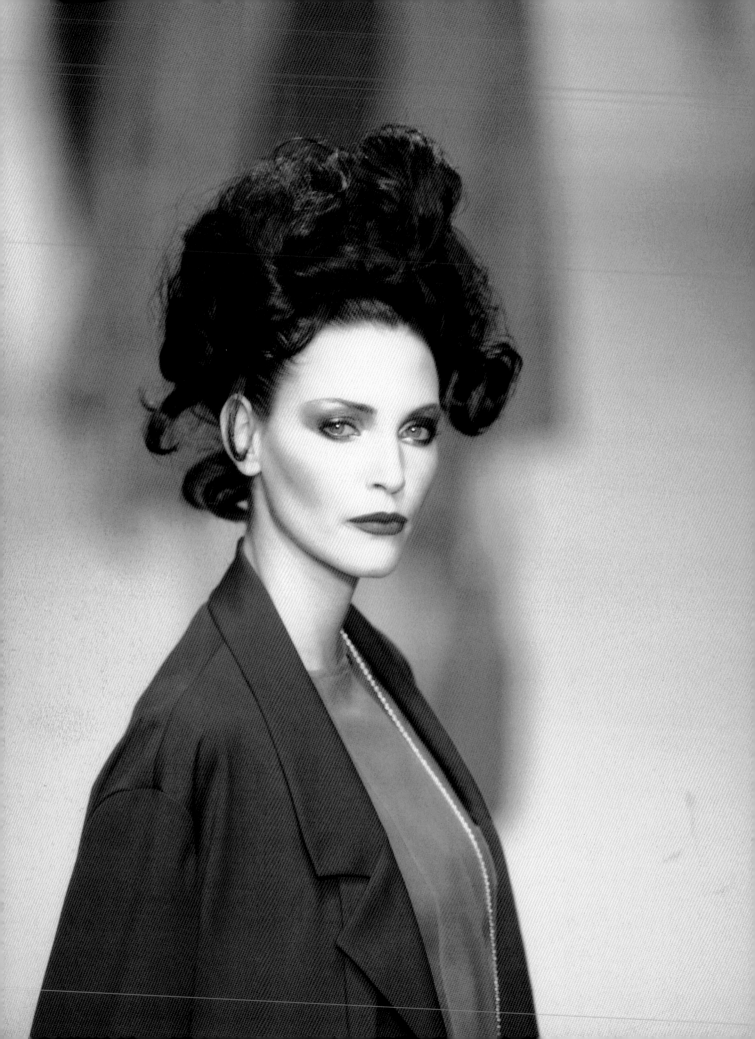

Karl Lagerfeld
Photograph © Niall McInerney

The majority of stylists today are self-employed and work across the board or are fashion editors employed full-time on magazines or newspapers.

In fashion, styling is crucial for editorial pages, runway shows, catalogues and advertising. Styling is vital in advertising campaigns for the launch of new products and also for the re-launch of old products which need to be re-directed to a new market or an existing consumer with whom the retailer has lost touch. By targeting a new and sophisticated consumer generation, a great stylist can resurrect the dinosaurs of design without losing touch with the philosophy of the retailer.

No one can be taught how to style and many fall into the role by accident. However most do have an art and design background. A successful stylist needs a passion for design, a good visual eye and a strong sense of colour and texture. There are many assets that will help someone get into the profession, the most important being great stamina. Physical and emotional strength may not be revealed on the pages of the glossy fashion magazines, but without these qualities even the most creative stylist will not be able to stay the course. For many stylists the most loathed part of the job is the lugging around of heavy suitcases, dress rails, kit bags and cumbersome props. The stylist is often the first to arrive and the last to leave a shoot and call times can be painfully early. Add to this long journeys to and from locations and working outdoors in the freezing cold or blistering heat – it is easy to see the need for stamina.

Many stylists find themselves working on trips abroad for most of the winter. In addition, attending the Paris, Milan, London and New York shows twice a year means weeks at a time away from home. Although this is inspiring and a great privilege, the novelty of travel can soon wear thin.

Photograph © John Akehurst

The stylist on a shoot has a great deal of responsibility. They answer to both the client and the photographer and are responsible not only for the clothes, accessories and props but also for the hair and make-up team and the models. Everything and everyone must be at the shoot, on time, in order for the job to be done well. Quite aside from the pressure to be creative, a tight budget, restricting brief and a fast-approaching deadline can add up to enormous stress for the stylist.

Team spirit and diplomacy are extremely important when working creatively with others under the pressures of time. The stylist without team spirit will find work tough going because of the need to discuss and accommodate other people's ideas and to get a result with which everyone is satisfied. Diplomacy is especially important when styling for a company whose philosophy is inflexible: the stylist needs the ability to second guess the client and know when to be forthcoming with ideas and when to take a step back.

In fashion and its related areas time is money, therefore punctuality is vital. A good stylist must have a totally organized approach to work and the ability to prioritize tasks and deal with the necessary paper work. The latter could be anything from a written or visual proposal to a budget or costing. Personal financing, like invoicing promptly, needs attention, and a cash flow facility may be necessary for buying props and accessories (some clients do not advance this money) so a good relationship with the bank is essential.

All stylists need to be aware of changing trends and attitudes. Developments in street style, music, television, film and the visual arts are as important to the stylist as trends and directions on the international runways. The successful stylist absorbs everything, from contemporary fashion, interior design, textiles and historical costume to changes in design, architecture, politics and youth culture, and uses it all as inspiration for great fashion stories.

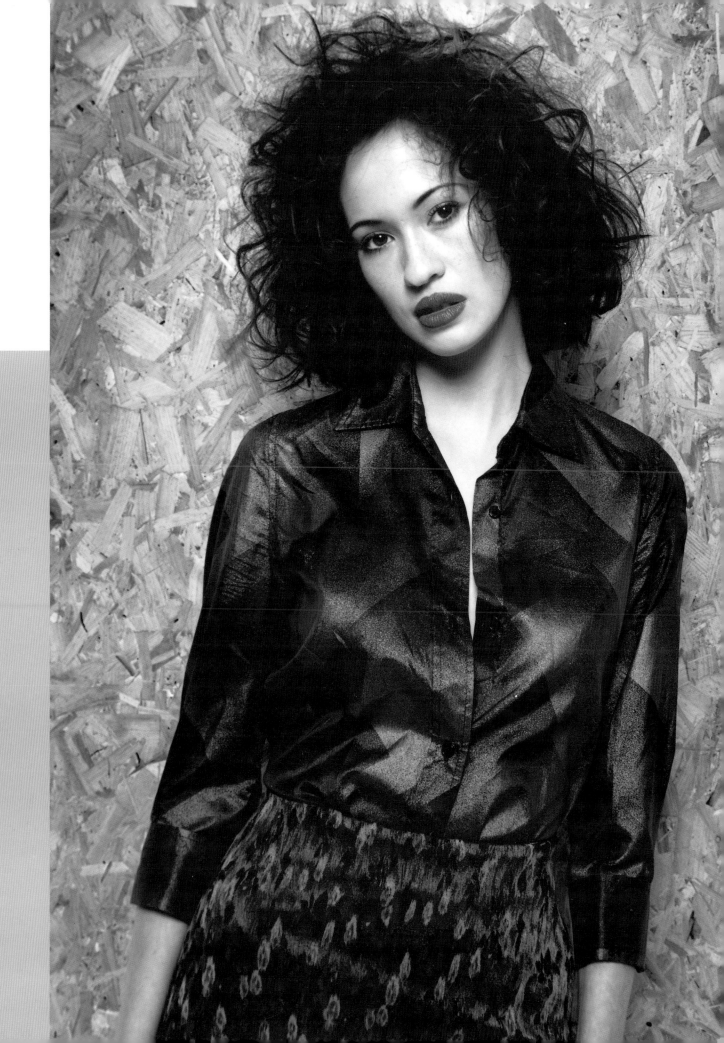

Photographer: Perry Ogden
Stylist: Alisa Green for French Connection

Would-be stylists learn their trade by assisting those who are experienced. It is an apprenticeship with a steep learning curve but, by being on shoots, working hard, looking, learning and making contacts within the industry, the transition from assistant to stylist need not take long.

Unless a stylist is employed full-time on a magazine or newspaper, most projects are commissioned on the basis of previous work. Stylists, like models, must keep a book (portfolio) of tear sheets (published editorial pages) to show to prospective clients as examples of their creativity and ability. Whilst assisting, most would-be stylists shoot test pictures with trainee photographers (often photographers' assistants whom they have met on shoots) and start a book of examples of their work with which they can secure an agent or their first jobs as fully-fledged stylists. The route to becoming a successful stylist can be made easier by being represented by a good agent. All agents take an agreed percentage and, in return, are responsible for sending out books to secure regular work and for negotiating and chasing payments. Agents help to reorganize the stylist's book so that it is concise and targets particular areas of fashion. It is advisable to have two portfolios: one more commercial, to help secure catalogue and advertising work, and another more creative, to demonstrate ability for editorial and runway styling. It is important that the prospective agent is sympathetic not only to the stylist's work but also to their needs and lifestyle.

There is no set method of working and the fledgling stylist will form a response to briefs that develops into their personal hallmark and the reason that they are offered work.

The relationship between the stylist and photographer is of paramount importance. Without a mutual understanding and response to the brief, the project in hand will seldom be a success. Therefore, stylists work with as many photographers as possible, learning from them along the way, and editing out those with whom the

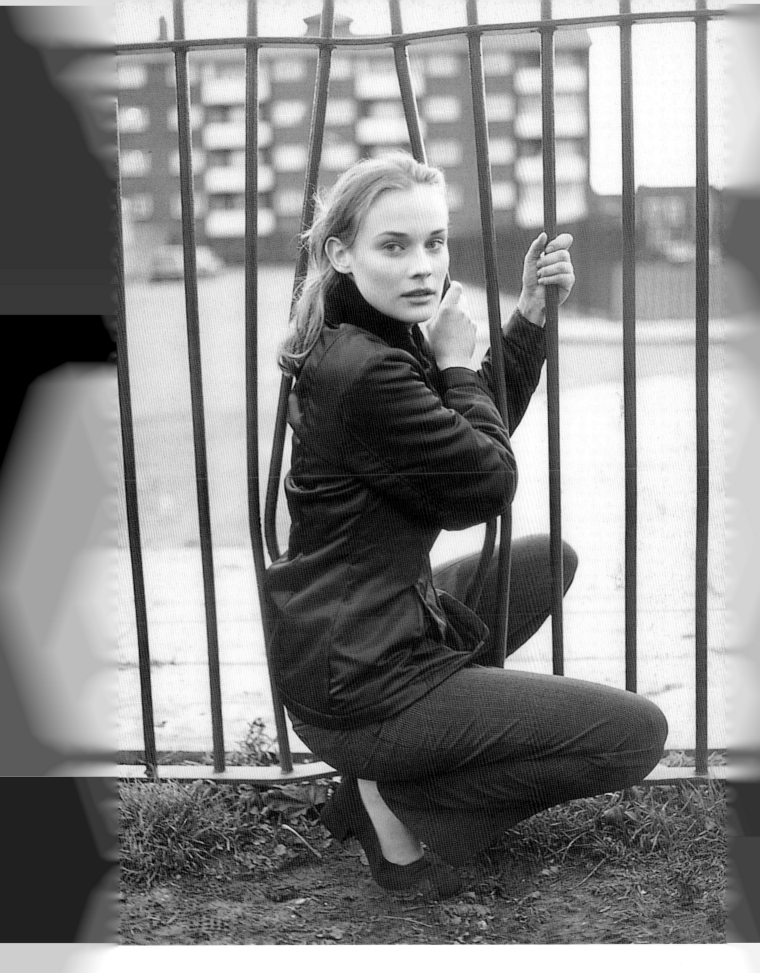

Photographer: Neil Kirk

Model: Helena Christensen for Dorothy Perkins

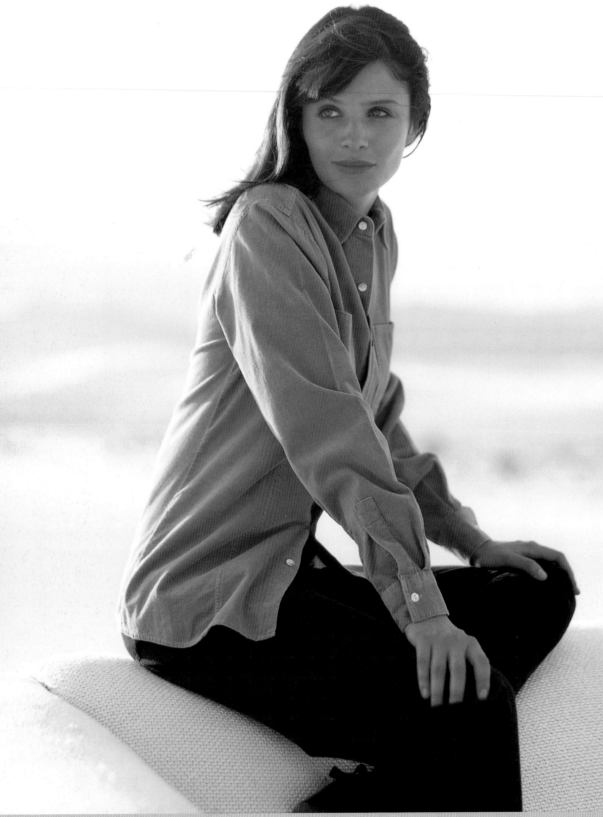

Photographer: Neil Kirk

Model: Helena Christensen for Dorothy Perkins

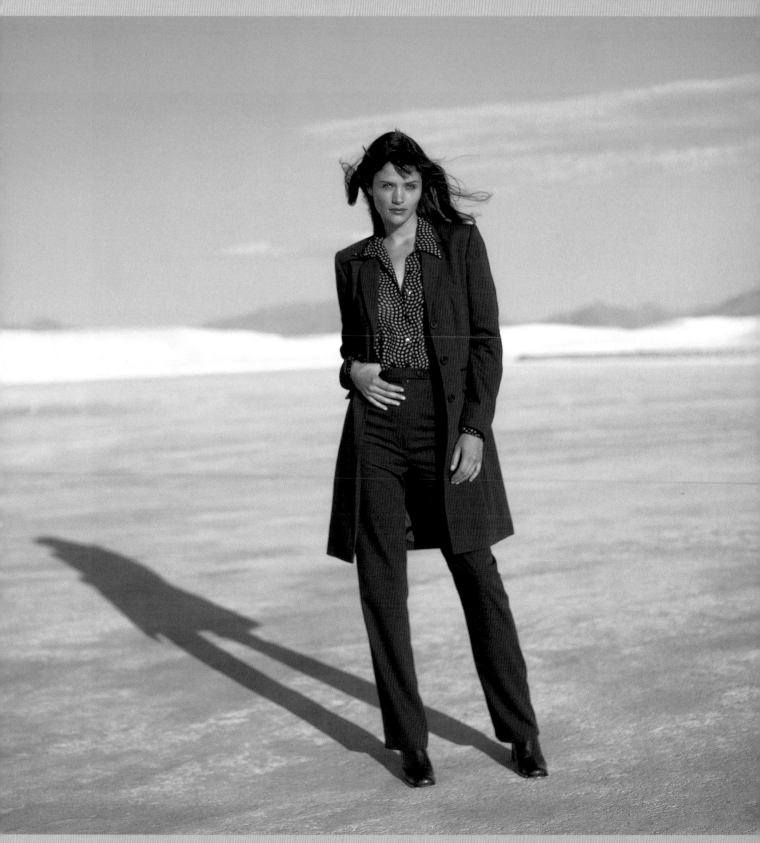

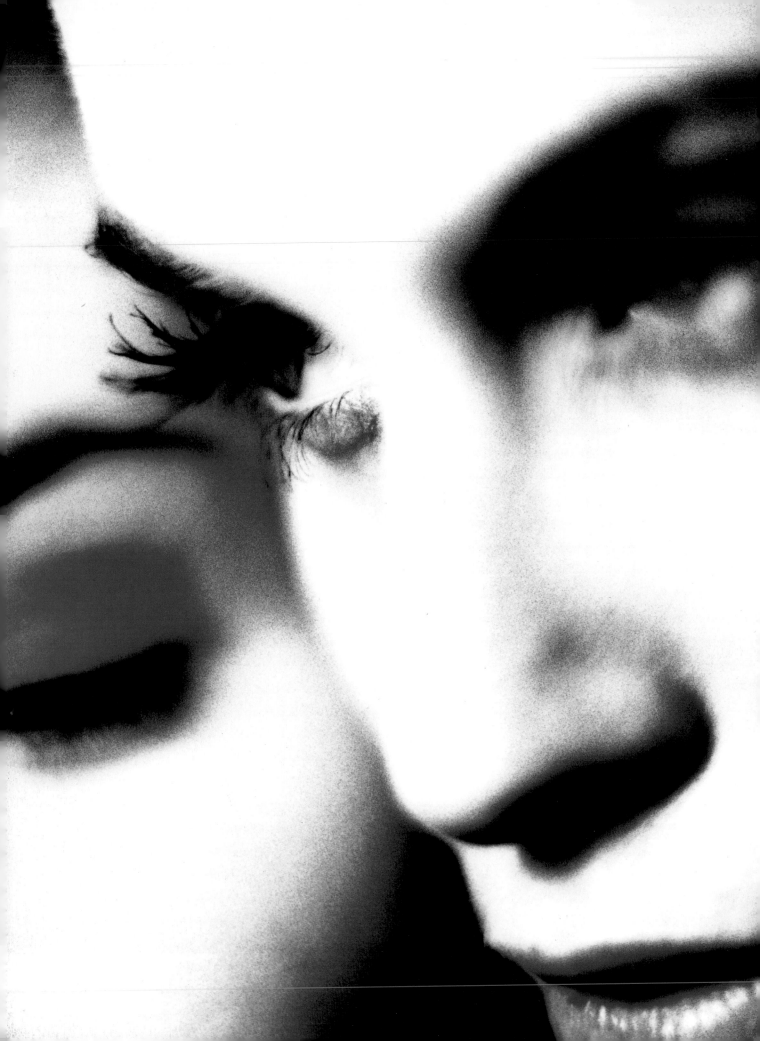

Photograph © Sandro Hyams

Make-Up: Carolee

Backstage

Photograph © Niall McInerney

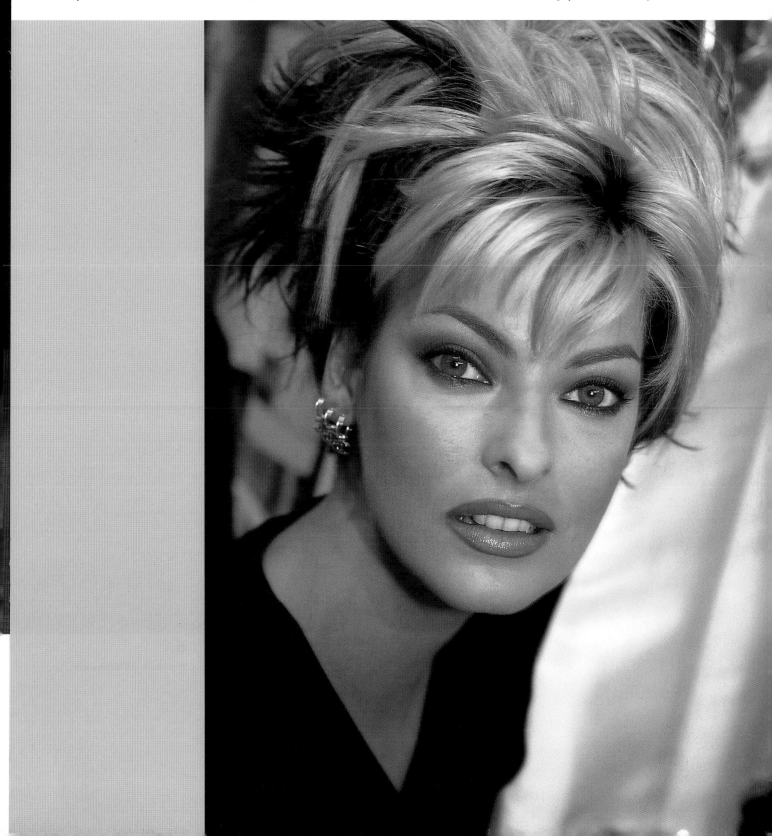

Runway stylists may specialize in this area or take time out from jobs at leading fashion magazines to work with designers during the collections - a rather prestigious bonus.

Apart from having a feel for the designer's work and the construction of clothes, the runway stylist must also comprehend how the show operates. For instance, unlike at a fashion shoot, where the number of models will often be limited to one, the show stylist will frequently be co-ordinating 4 or 5 outfits for each of 20 or more models. Ideas are one thing but equally important is to follow through the finer details of a vast number of outfits. Before the show, the stylist views the collection and plans the accessories. Shoes, jewellery and millinery are normally borrowed for a credit, hired for a fee or specially designed by an accessory designer and paid for. The stylist is usually responsible for sourcing all accessories. For example, if the designer agrees that sheer hosiery will be worn with every outfit throughout the show, it is the stylist's task to make sure a pair is allocated to each and every outfit.

Deciding on the running order - the order in which the outfits appear on the runway - is a collaboration between the designer, stylist and show producer. The stylist can advise as to which garments are worn together to form outfits and can suggest the addition of key garments they feel the collection lacks. A runway show stylist will be expected to input suggestions for models. It is important to be up-to-date with the important new faces in modelling and to know whose look will complement the collection and which models will generate publicity pictures. It is preferable for each model to try on their outfits in advance, either on the day of the show, or, if they are available, during the days leading up to the show. All outfits allocated should fit correctly and suit the models. This process is overseen by the stylist and, if there are problems with fit, the stylist provides the solutions, either by getting the design team to make alterations or by trying the outfit on another model.

The collection may be divided into sub-sections or themes that follow the overall look of the collection, but the styling and accessories will differ slightly to be

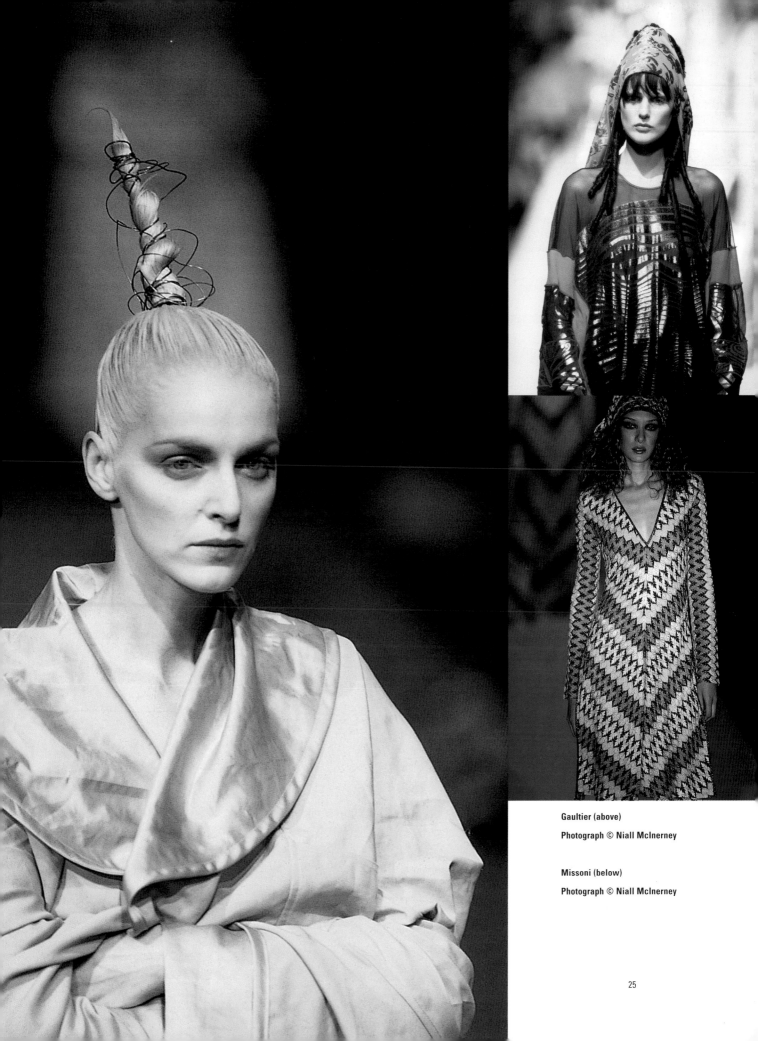

Gaultier (above)
Photograph © Niall McInerney

Missoni (below)
Photograph © Niall McInerney

25

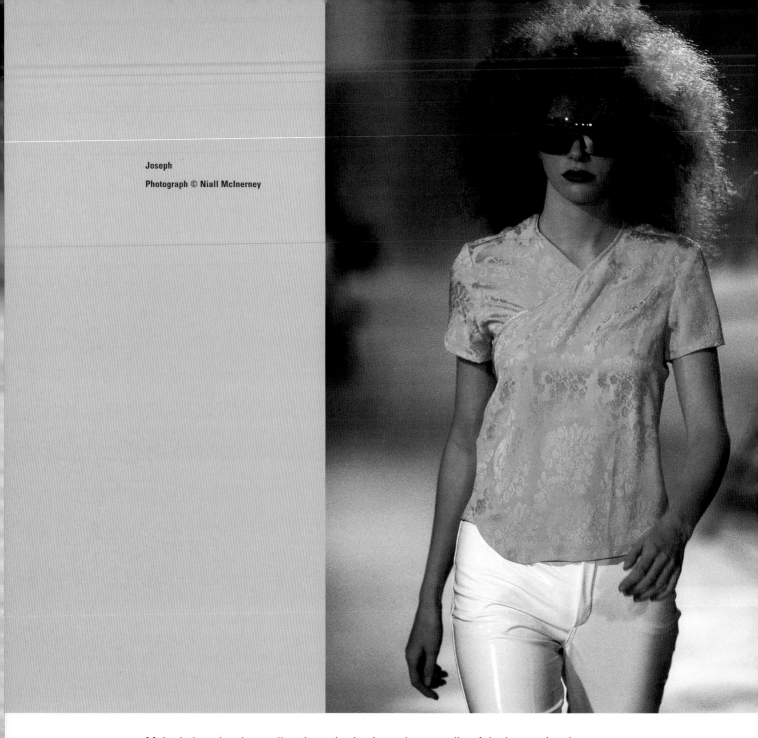

Joseph
Photograph © Niall McInerney

Major hair and make-up directions also begin on the catwalks of the international ready-to-wear collections. The hair and make-up image-makers chosen by international designers are becoming the new fashion personalities and are enjoying as much media attention as the designers that employ them and the models on which they work.

Runway shows are one of the most creative areas for hair and make-up artists, especially when working for big name designers during the ready-to-wear collections. Here they can bring a touch of extravagance to the show, or, if the styling of the collection is pared down and minimal, they can give the overall look a new direction.

Galliano
Photograph © Niall McInerney

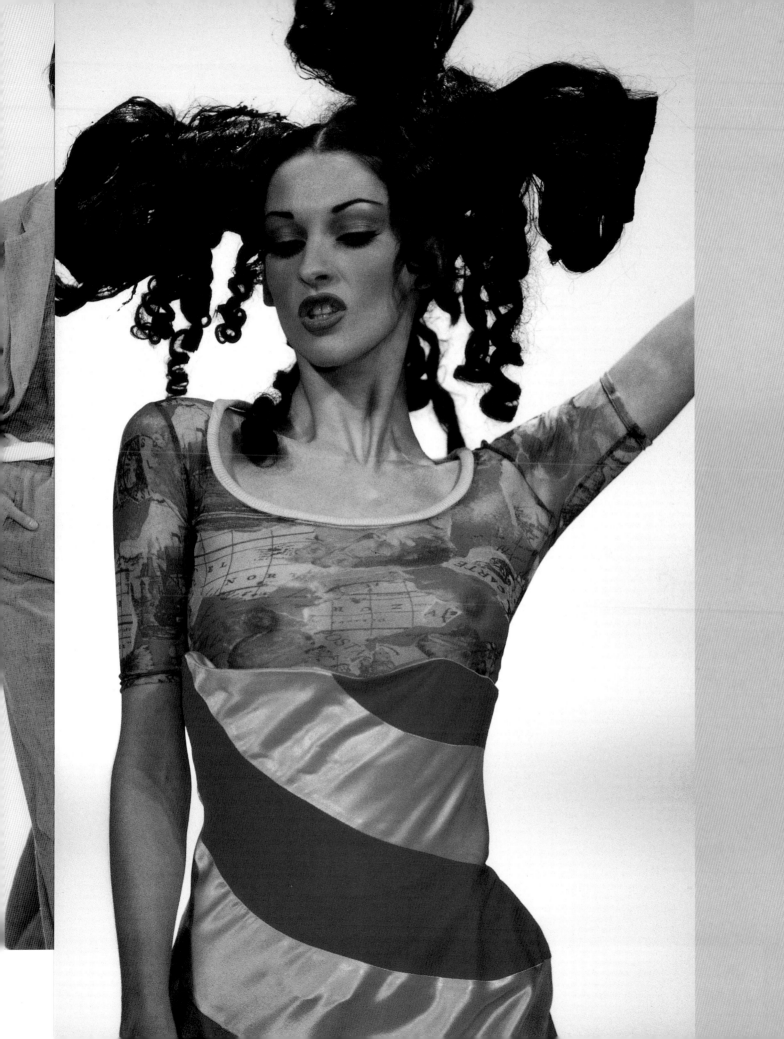

Comme des Garçons

Photograph © Niall McInerney

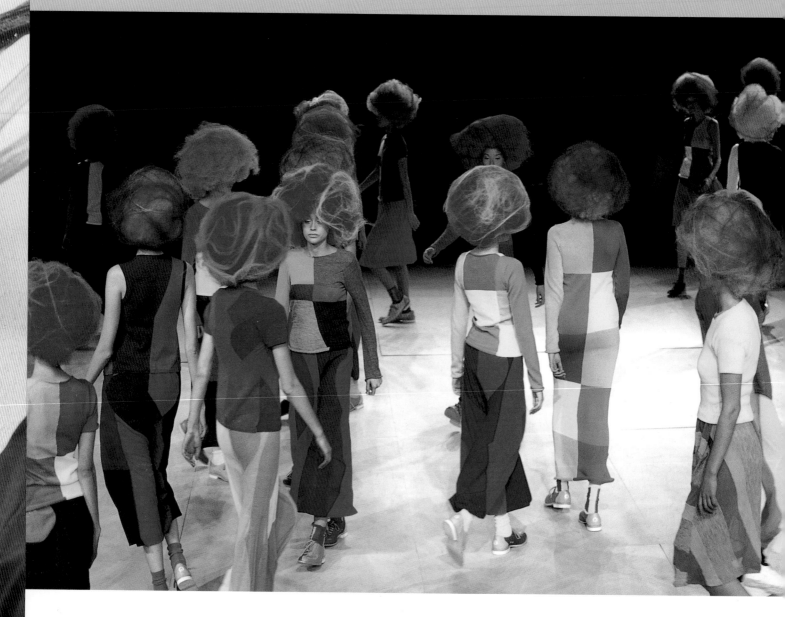

Designers choose a hair and make-up team who will complement the collection.
It is important that the team is sympathetic to the styling, but equally, the designer
and the stylist should understand the work of different hair and make-up teams so
that the right people are booked for the job.

Often working in pairs, the hair and make-up duo create high-profile, influential
looks that break new ground. Eventually these will not only be seen in editorial
shoots, but will also become an inspiration for the whole fashion and beauty
industry, from teen mags to fashion ad campaigns to influencing the seasonal
make-up palettes of the major cosmetic companies. As with fashion directions,

Hussein Chalayan
Photograph © Niall McInerney

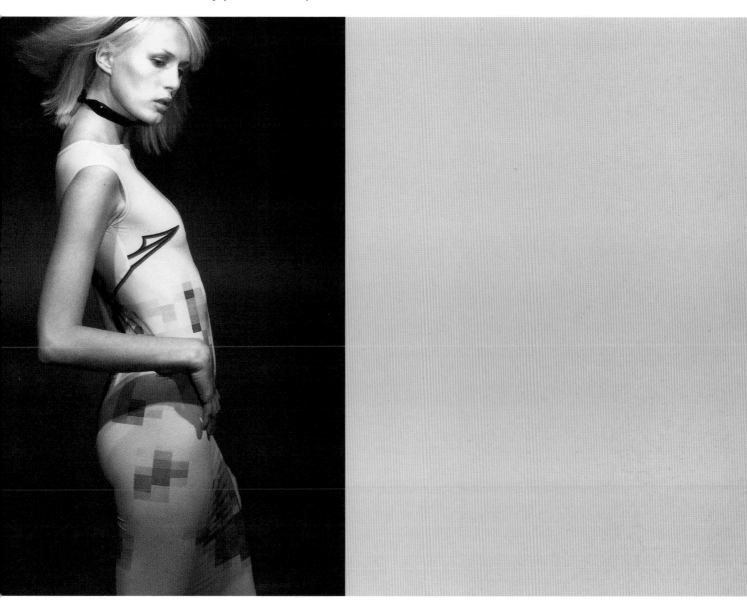

make-up looks change continually, from natural 'no make-up make-up', shimmer, metallics and pearlized effects to glamorous, bright and vibrant colours.

Ideally, the hair stylist and make-up artist see sketches or Polaroids of the collection weeks before the show, at worst, the day before or on the show day. When the collection has been seen, the hair and make-up team will start creating ideas. They may liaise with each other so that a total look is created for the runway. They may sketch or use tear sheets as reference and do make-up try outs on models that they know will be used in the show. It is especially important that hair 'fittings' take place if more outrageous or complicated hair styles are to be created.

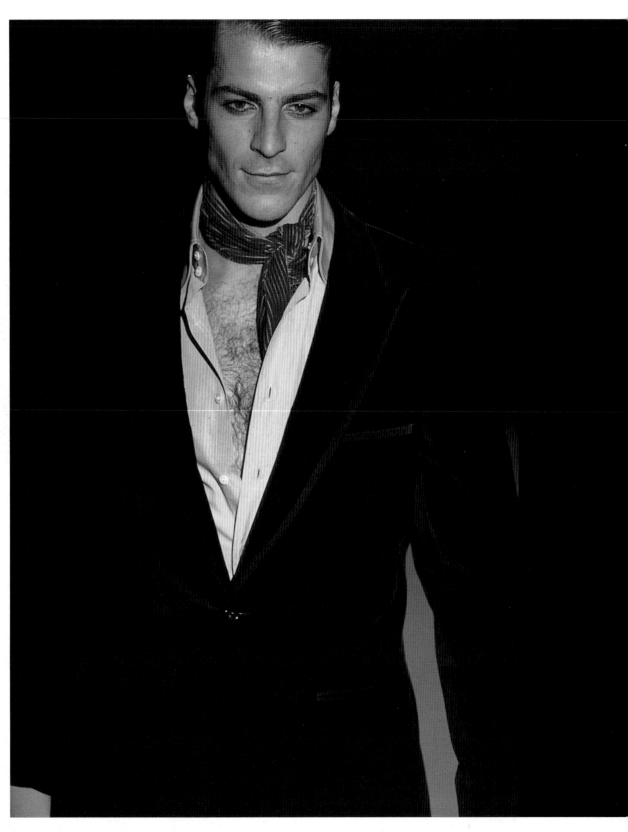

Gucci

Photograph © **Niall McInerney**

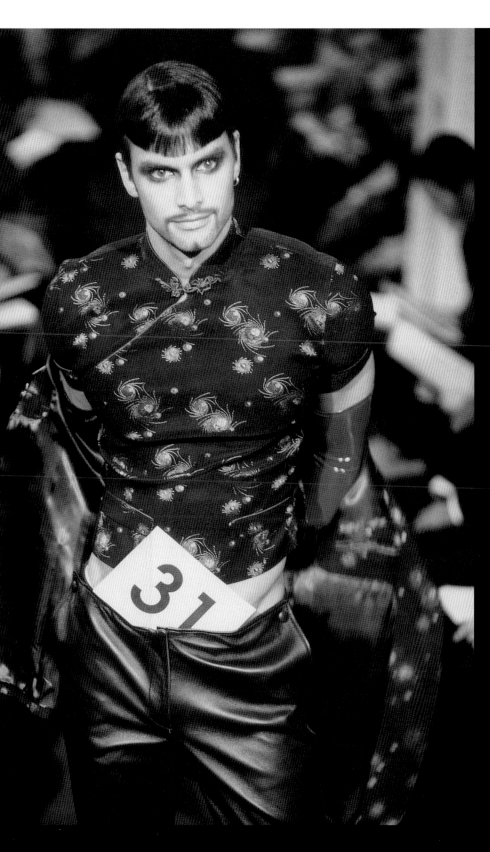

Gaultier

Photograph © Niall McInerney

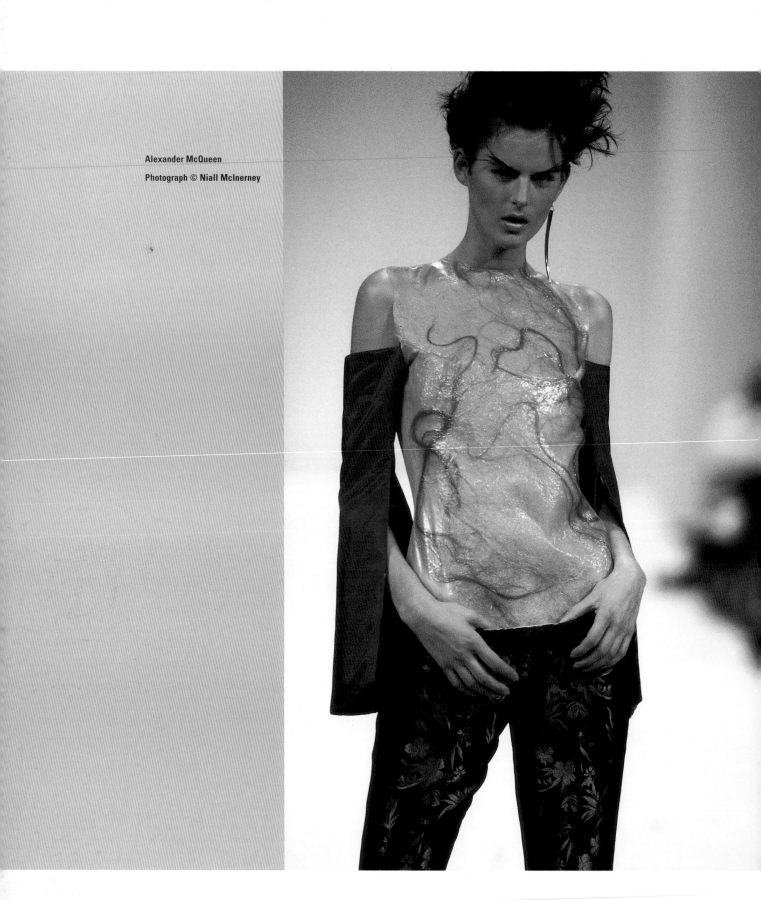

Alexander McQueen

Photograph © Niall McInerney

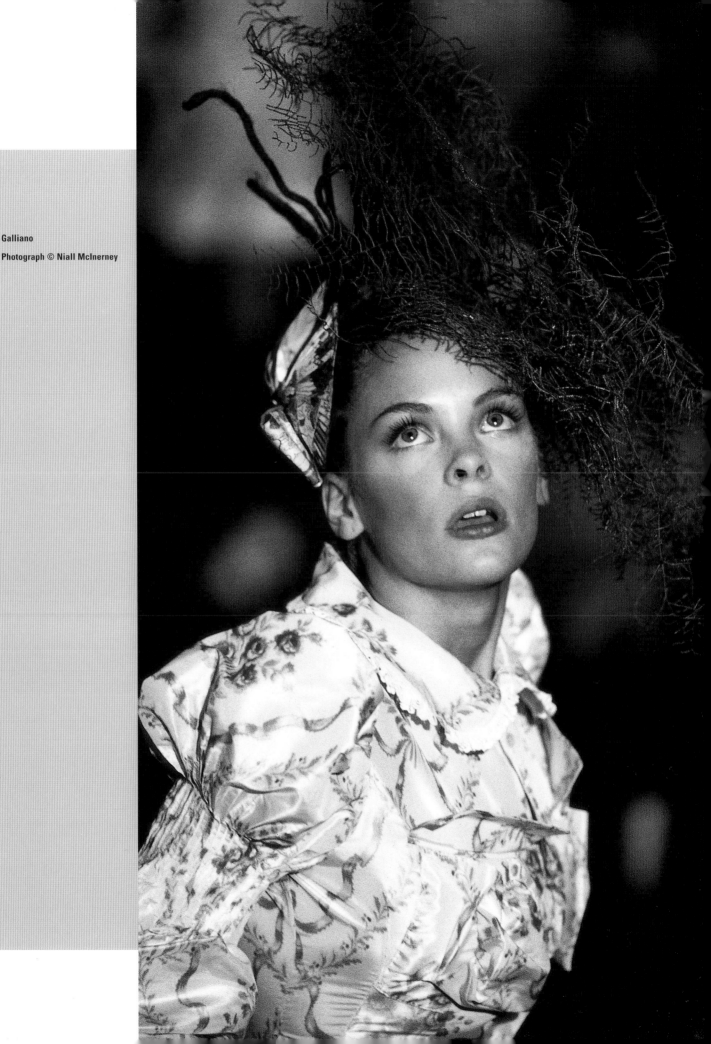

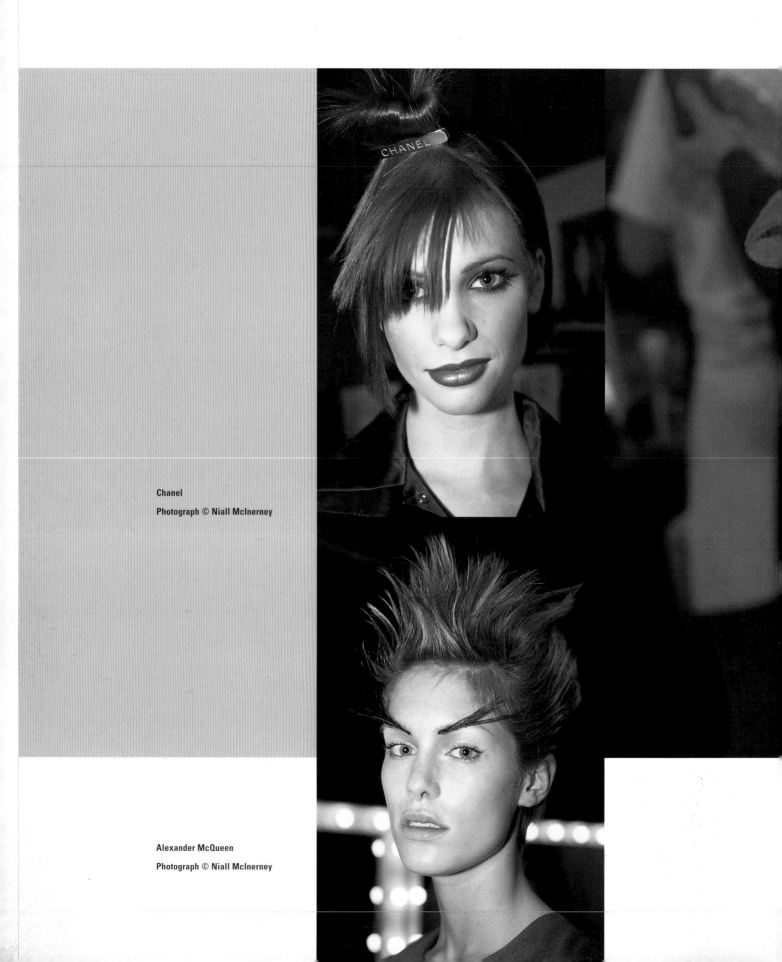

Chanel

Photograph © Niall McInerney

Alexander McQueen

Photograph © Niall McInerney

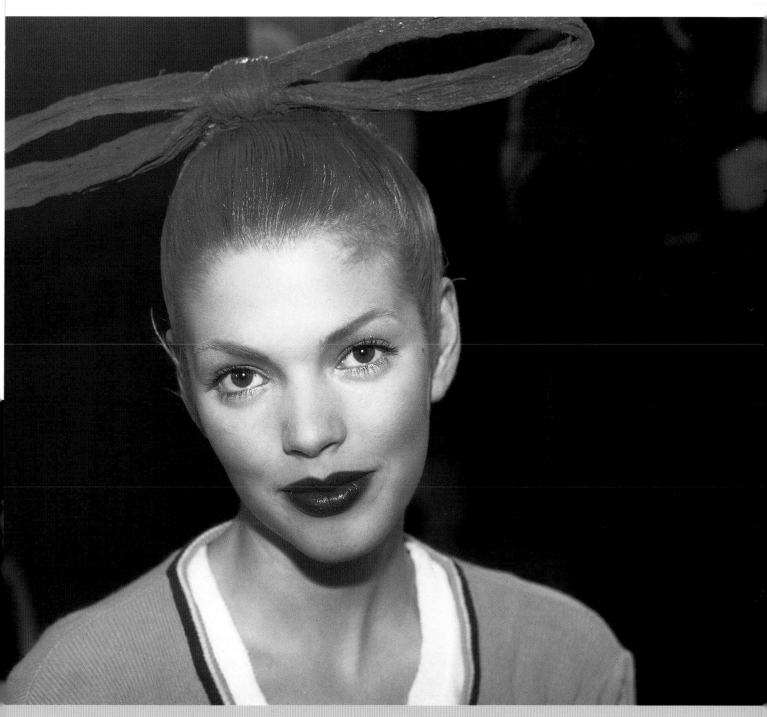

Givenchy

Photograph © Niall McInerney

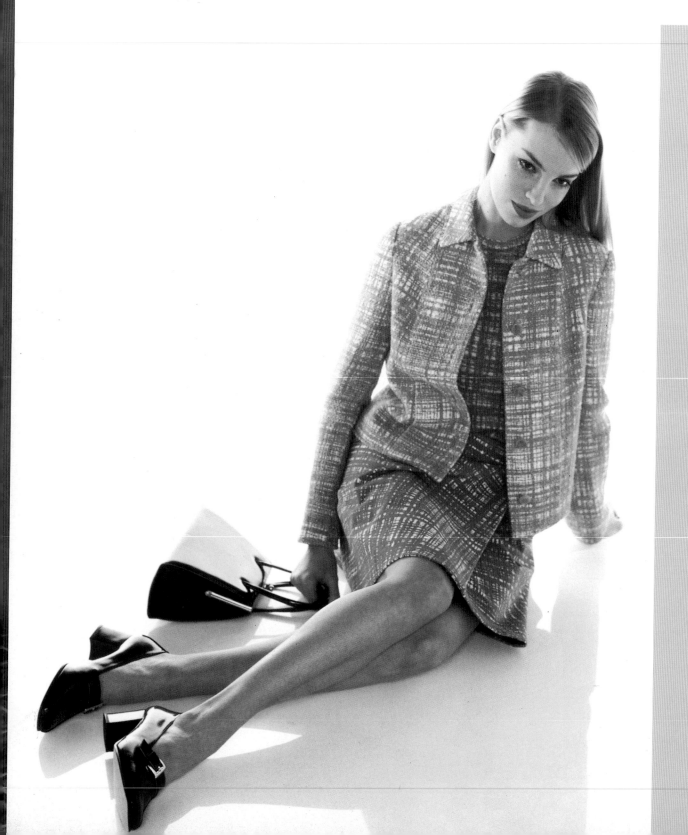

When the final show of the season is over, fashion directors, editors and stylists set about deciding which of the new fashion directions are the most important. Fashion editors will ignore certain directions that do not suit the feel of their particular magazine, opting for those that best reflect the style of their publication and their readers' attitude.

Magazines may have fashion editors on their staff who style all the fashion stories themselves but some fashion editors may be given a budget for commissioning freelance stylists for one-off editorial stories.

Once the fashion themes to be covered have been agreed, they are allocated to the stylist. The stylist thinks up the visual story that best reflects the theme and decides which photographer would best complement the story by looking at new photographers' books and considering those with whom they have worked before. This is an enormously creative process as, within limits, the editorial stylist has complete control of the pages. Once the photographer is on board, dates for shooting are set and the process of choosing models and locations begins. Being open to suggestions from the photographer and art director is a creative process in itself, as a fresh eye and new twists can really open up a story. Most magazines have a page rate, a budget that must be adhered to, and every cost from transport to model fees must be included. Generally, more pages filled with one shoot means more budget to play with overall.

To find the right model or models it may be necessary for the photographer and stylist to hold a casting. If so, the model agencies are contacted, the story and the type of model needed is explained and models arrive at the magazine with their books for the stylist and photographer to choose from. Again, the stylist must be up-to-date with new faces on the modelling scene and have good contacts with the major international model agencies. Both the stylist and photographer must agree on the kind of model that suits the magazine and the story to be shot. A short list is made and the models are optioned. The model agency will give a first option,

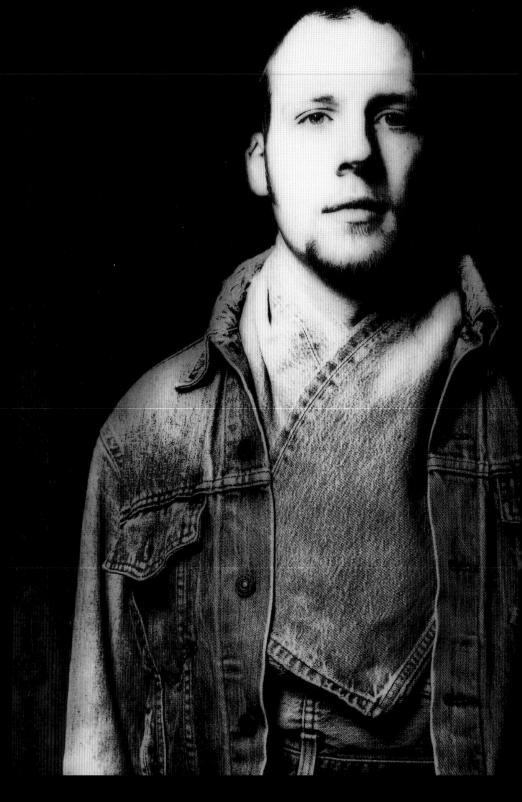

Editorial

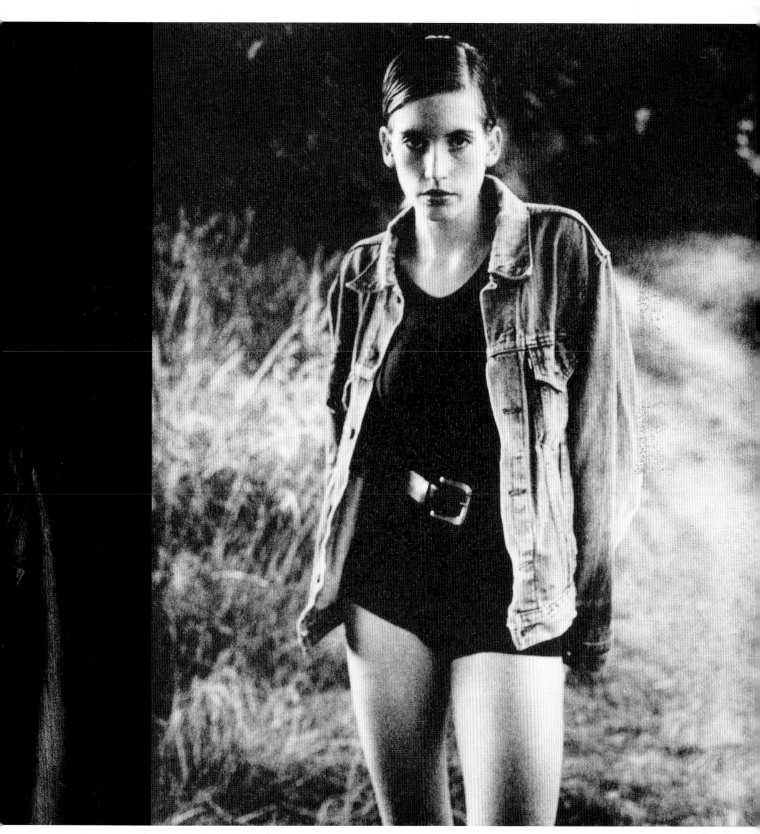

Photograph © Chris Denehy

Photograph © Richard Truscott

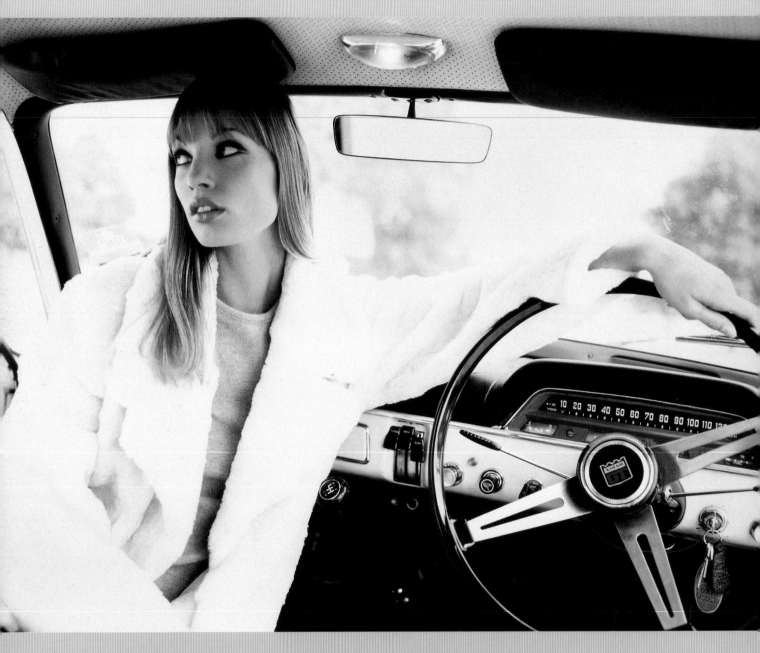

meaning first refusal, or a second option, meaning someone else holds the first
option. Only if they decide not to confirm will the second option change to the much
coveted first. When this happens, the model can be confirmed, in writing, giving
call times, location addresses and an outline of fees.

The photographer may book a studio or recce locations, bringing back Polaroids
for approval. If the location is abroad, research is done from visual references.
The location and models are approved by the fashion director or magazine editor.

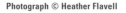

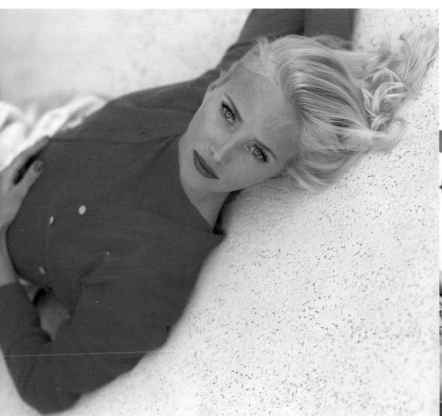 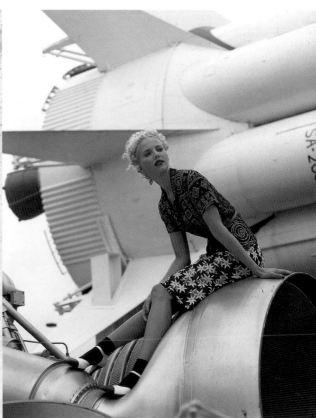

At the same time, the stylist sets about selecting suitable clothes and accessories, either by visiting PR agencies who hold sample ranges of high street brands and designer collections or by referring to notes made during previous PR agency open days or designer runway shows. Editorial fashion is about clothing that is available to the reader during the time the issue of the magazine or newspaper is on the newstands. Clothing that is unavailable to buy is discouraged by magazine editors as the purpose of the fashion pages is to offer fashion ideas and sources that are accessible to the reader. The stylist keeps this in mind when selecting. The clothes are sent in to the magazine by the PR. The stylist then makes a further edit on what has arrived, whittling down the garments and putting together outfits until the required number has been selected. Most stylists put together more outfits than are necessary in case something does not look right on the day of the shoot.

The stylist and photographer choose a hair stylist and make-up artist by looking through books requested from agencies. Obviously they look for capability and talent but also for something that shows sympathy to the theme of the story. They also consider personality, as no amount of talent can make up for people who are difficult to work with. The optioning system is the same as that for models, so a short list of names is optioned and when firsts become available, hair and make-up are confirmed.

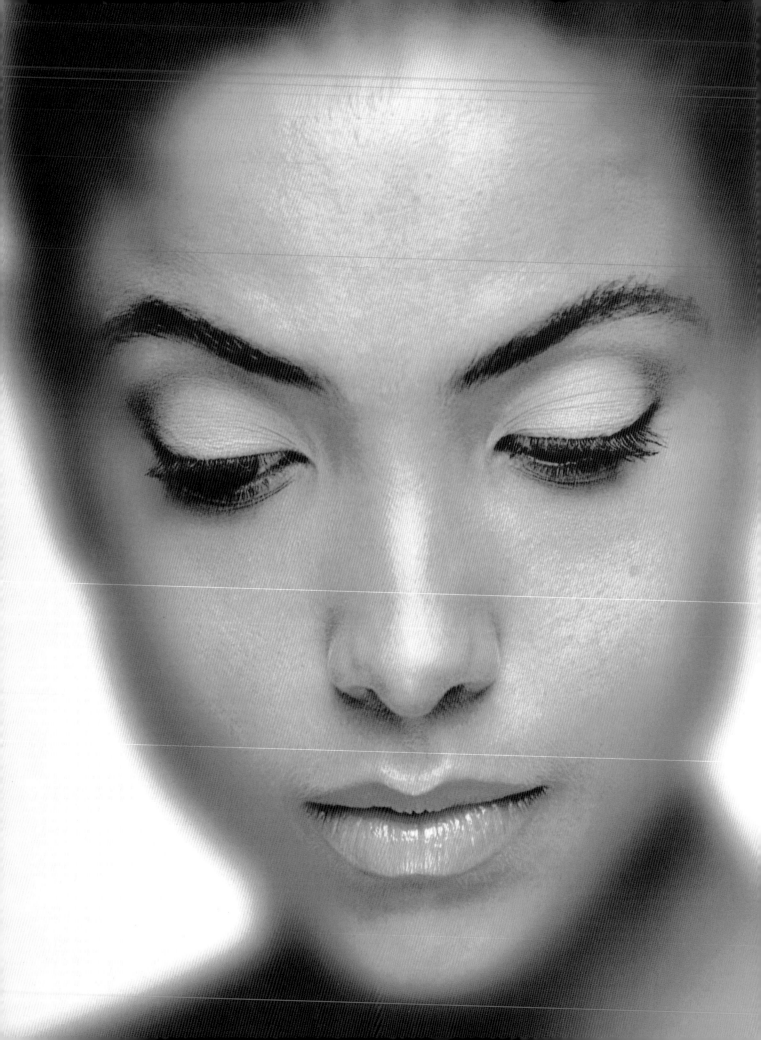

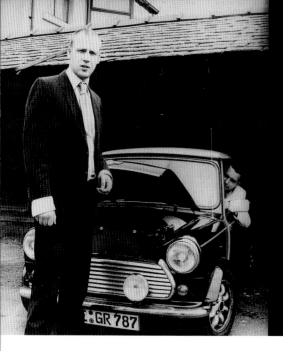

Photograph © Chris Denehy

A stylist working full-time on a magazine is a commisioning editor and, in the case of editorial shoots, is therefore the client. The team take their direction from the stylist who thus shoulders the responsibility for the whole shoot.

Logistically, the studio is the easiest place to shoot, though it is an empty shell and can limit the variety of shots. Locations offer more range and realism to a shoot but mean working out of a cramped location van and dealing with the weather conditions. Trips abroad involve travelling with heavy suitcases full of clothes and accessories, coping with travel and accommodation arrangements, location recces, long days and possible adverse weather conditions.

The stylist on an editorial shoot follows a certain working pattern, whether in a studio, on location or abroad on a trip. When the model arrives, outfits are tried on and a final clothes' edit is made and communicated to the photographer. A shooting order of outfits is then decided and, after a briefing and a look through the clothes, hair and make-up begin. This gives the stylist a chance to press, steam and prepare the outfits which are then hung on a dress rail in the order in which they will be shot.

Once the model is dressed, a Polaroid is taken on set for the team to check. When everyone is satisfied, shooting on film begins and the stylist, hair stylist and make-up artist watch the model, intervening as and when adjustments are needed. The process is repeated until all the clothes have been shot. A Polaroid of each outfit is taken and these can be used by the magazine art director, if present, or by the stylist and photographer to crop and mock up the page layout as the shoot progresses.

Once back at the magazine, the stylist waits for the film to come in from the photographer. They edit it with the magazine art director, marking the shots that they think work the best. Using a loop, they look for all-round satisfactory shots, then, check that there are no minute flaws that will show upon the printed page.

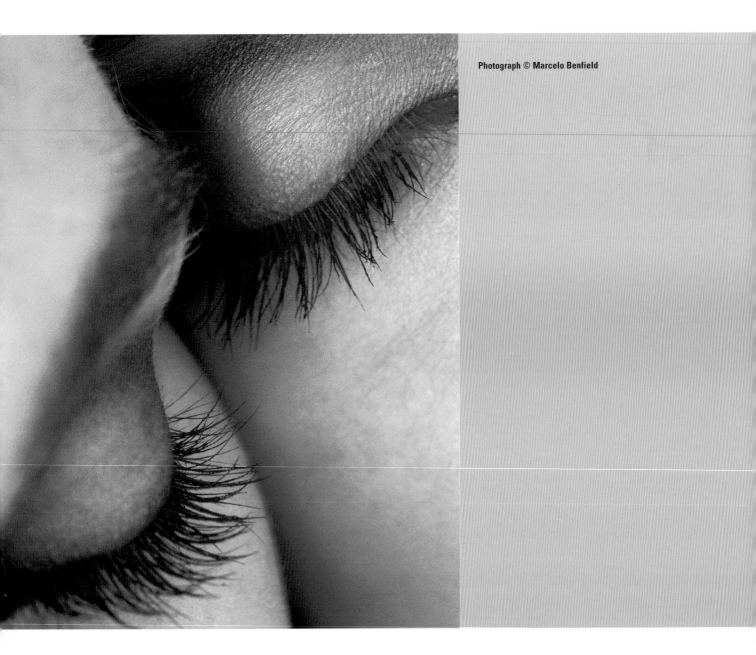

Photograph © Marcelo Benfield

The pictures are passed to the art department to be laid out. The stylist sets to work, returning the clothes to the PRs and carefully documenting all returns as proof that everything has gone back to the right place. Prices and stockists for each garment are requested from the PR and captioned on each page of the story. Credits for the photographer, stylist, hair stylist, make-up artist and model are added. The proofs are then checked and corrected and once the magazine editor has passed the pages and the art director has approved the Cromalins, the pages go to press.

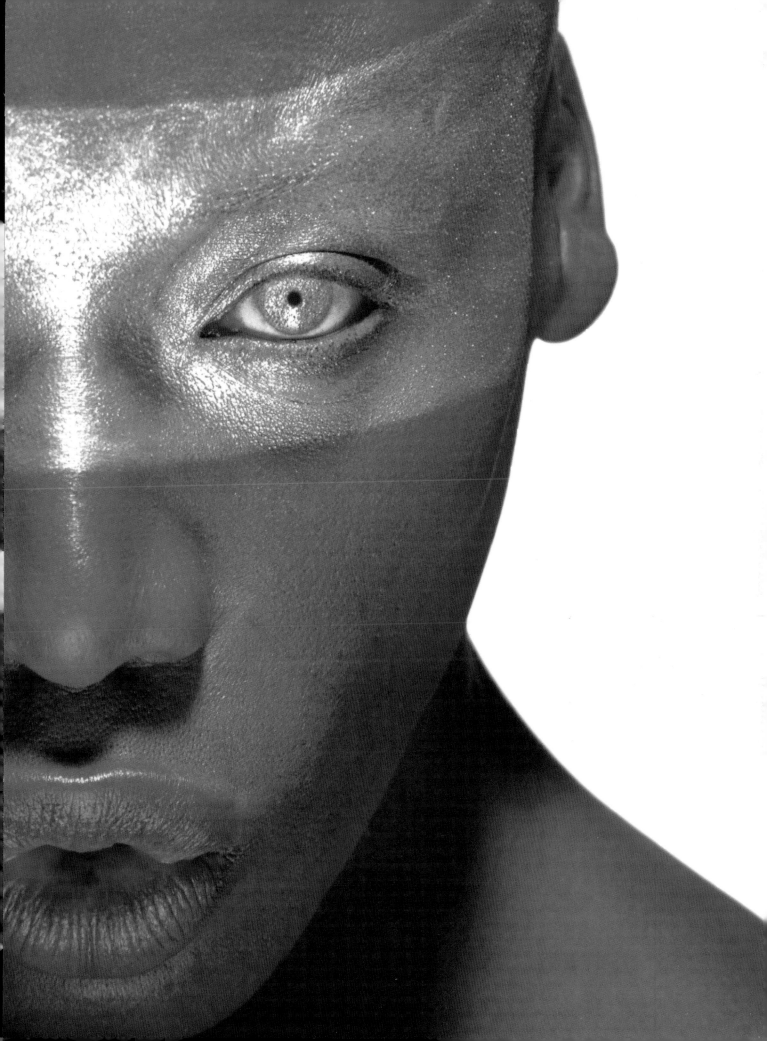

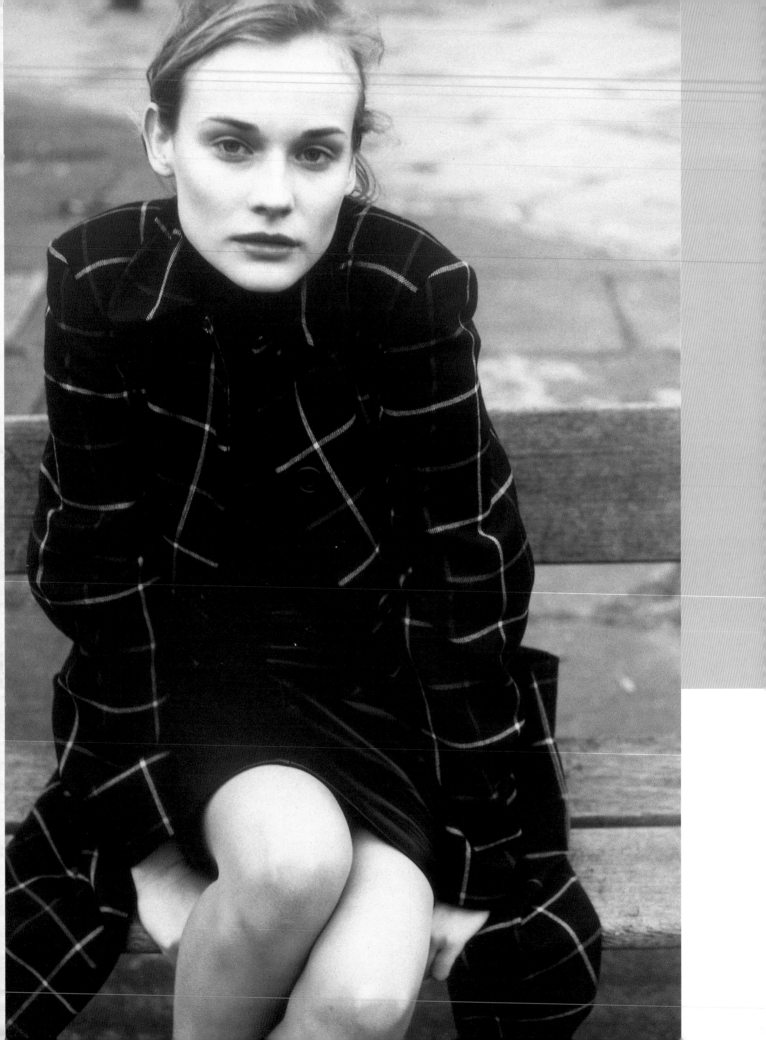

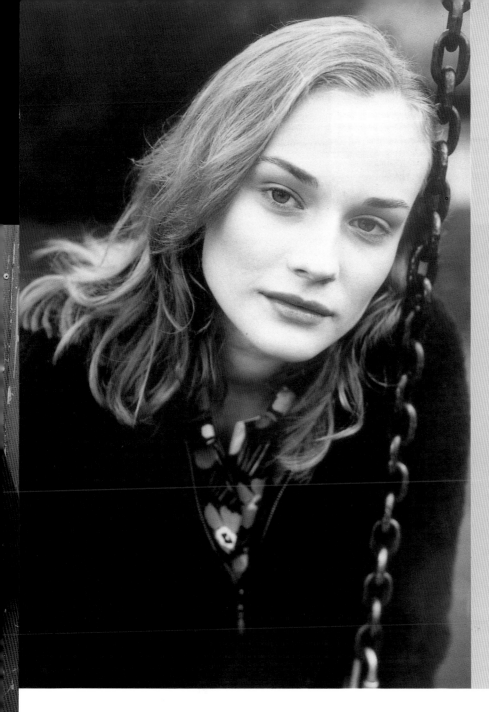

Photographer: Perry Ogden

Stylist: Alisa Green for French Connection

For stylists, hair stylists and make-up artists, creative control is limited, but advertising is where the money is.

The stylist is chosen by the advertising agency on behalf of the fashion client and therefore will not have the creative control that they would expect on an editorial job. Advertising briefs vary in flexibility from client to client. Clients wishing to launch or re-launch a fashion brand may want the stylist to act as consultant on a total brand concept, in which case the job is loaded with creative input and responsibility. This is hugely satisfying, and demands a thorough understanding of the brand, its target consumer and the market competition. Here the role of stylist overlaps with that of the art director and is a new area for successful stylists to explore.

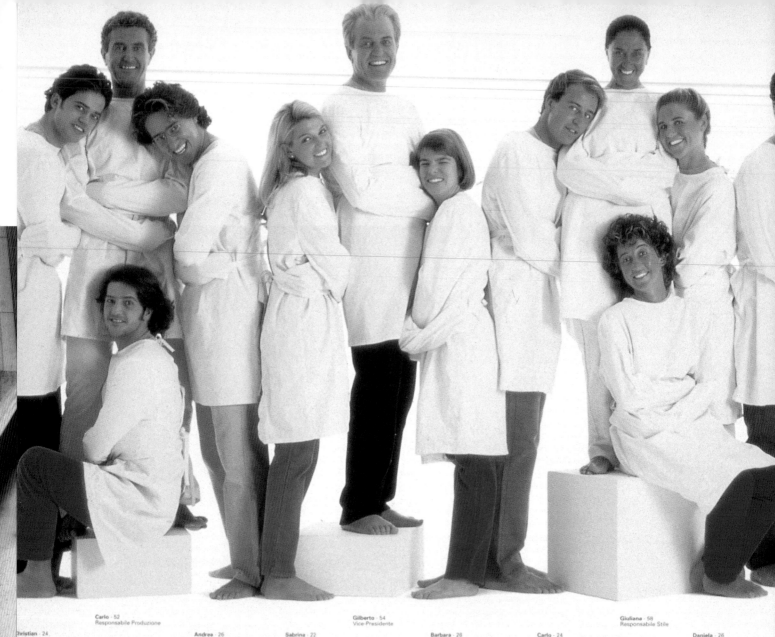

Carlo · 52
Responsabile Produzione

Gilberto · 54
Vice-Presidente

Giuliana · 58
Responsabile Stile

Christian · 24
Studente

Andrea · 26
Studente

Sabrina · 22
Studentessa

Barbara · 26
Studentessa

Carlo · 24
Consulente Finanziario

Daniela · 26
Progetto Undercolors

Massimo · 28
Studente

Paola · 37
Responsabile Prodotto

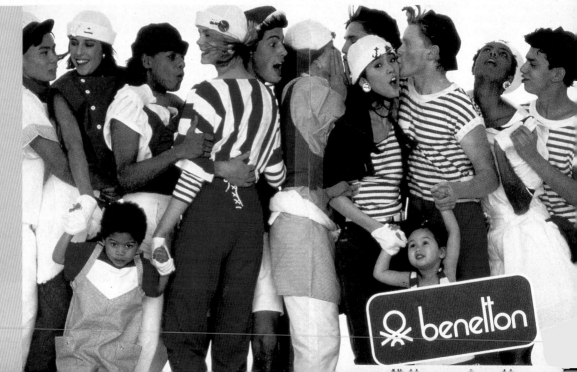

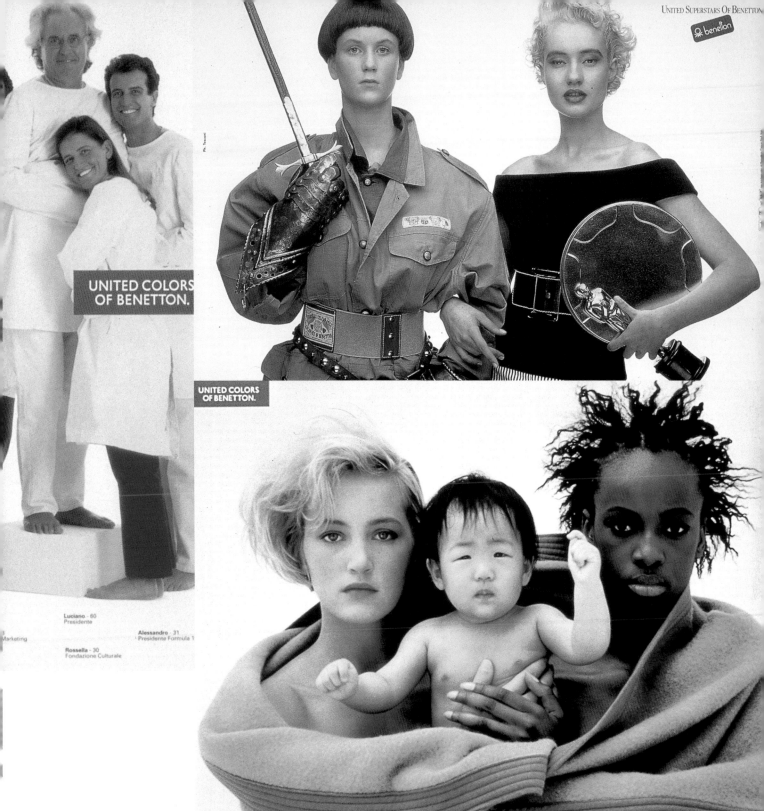

UNITED COLORS OF BENETTON.

UNITED COLORS OF BENETTON.

Luciano - 60
Presidente

Marketing

Alessandro - 31
Presidente Formula 1

Rossella - 30
Fondazione Culturale

Photographer: Toscani for Benetton

61

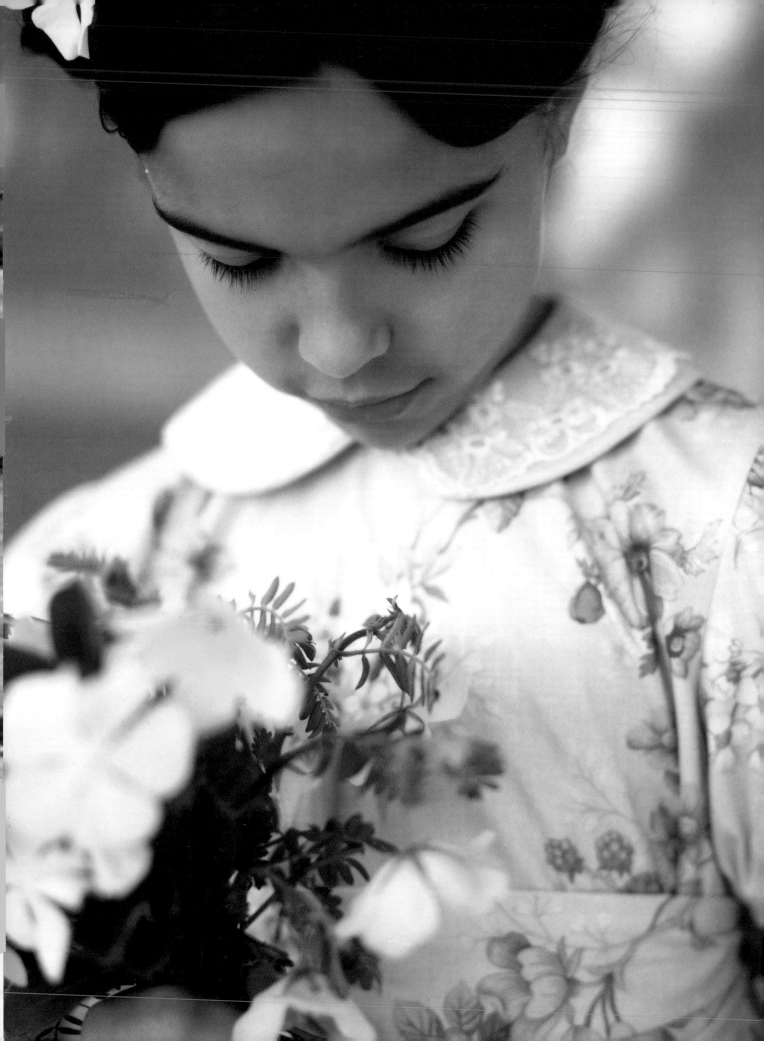

Catalogue

Many stylists say that working for catalogues is one of the toughest areas of their work. The purpose of catalogues is to sell products off the page, therefore only clothing and accessories that are available for the consumer to purchase can be used in the shots. This limitation puts an emphasis on the creativity of hair styling, make-up and propping. The wide consumer target means that the shots, whilst being aspirational, must remain simple and accessible. The emphasis is on the art direction – the marriage of image and type – to make the pages succeed.

Photographer: Stefano Azario

Stylist: Helen Crowther

Art Direction: Davies Baron for Mothercare UK Ltd

Photographer: Eamon McCabe for Next Directory

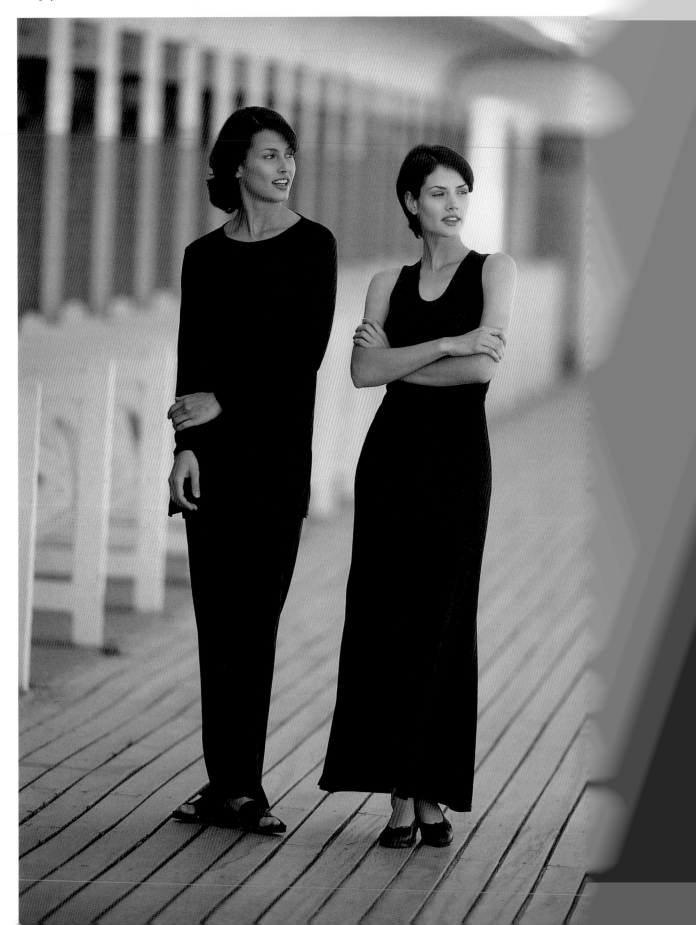

Generally, catalogues sell mass-market clothing to a consumer who wants high fashion at low prices. The task of the stylist is to make the clothes look perfect, to ensure that the correct garment details are highlighted, to prop the shots and to direct successful hair and make-up.

Once booked for a catalogue the stylist and photographer meet the art director and are briefed on the feel that should be achieved through the photography. At this meeting, the art director talks through the layouts which have been drawn up specifically and are the blue prints for the photographic shoot. The layouts explain how the garments will appear, the number of shots per page, the shape of each shot and where the copy will fall, so setting the parameters to which the team must work. The clothing is usually presented to the stylist by the buyer or design team for that particular clothing section. They will explain the inspiration behind the designs and will have ideas about how they see the garments being shot.

Once the garments have been seen and the client's opinions expressed, the stylist looks at accessories and comes up with ideas for styling and propping, models, hair and make-up team and locations. The stylist is responsible for taking notes at the briefing on behalf of the whole team. Usually the team will be working on one section of the catalogue at a time. The overall styling of each section must work within the theme of the whole and not jump out of character. The creativity here is to use styling ideas that work within the set boundaries.

The total number of shots expected by the client on a catalogue shoot usually outnumbers that for any other kind of shoot. As catalogue shoots are often abroad for a number of days, the schedule is gruelling.

Once abroad, the photographer, client and stylist recce suitable locations and work out a shooting schedule for each day of the trip. The stylist allocates time for prop sourcing and buying as there will not be enough time for this once shooting begins. Models are either flown in for the shoot, if they have been previously cast, or cast

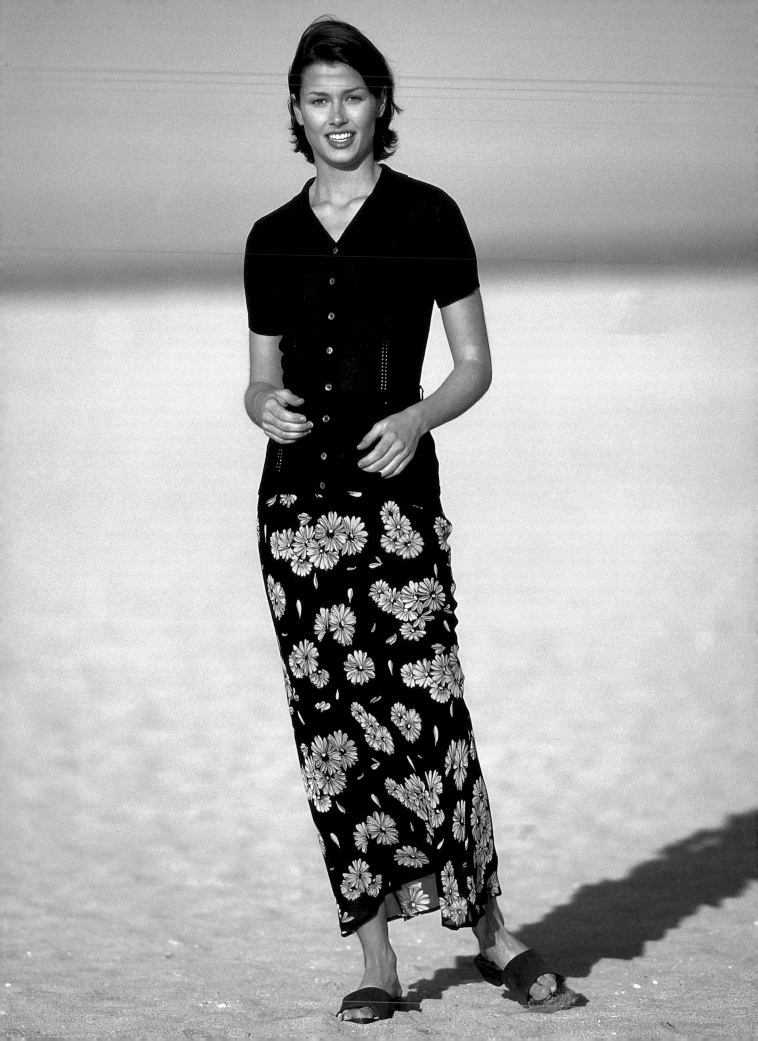

Photographer: Graham Montgomery for Next Directory

from local agencies. If local agencies are available, then castings need to be organized and models optioned and confirmed in the usual manner. Time for this will need to be allocated. On big trips, a production company may be contracted to organize castings, transport and locations. Once models, locations and shooting schedule are confirmed, and this information has been communicated to the whole team, shooting begins. Every evening the stylist must put away the clothing from the day's shooting and prepare the clothes for the next. The shoot days follow the usual structure and, as with advertising, it is vital that the client is happy at every stage. They should be offered Polaroids for approval and the art director will work with the stylist and photographer to ensure that the layout is followed. In hot locations, shooting starts early to use the valuable time before the midday sun gets too bright for pictures. When this happens, the shoot moves into the shade to continue or takes a break and recommences when the sun has cooled. After a late finish, using the last of the sun, and preparing tomorrow's clothes, the evenings on this kind of trip generally mean entertaining the client and the rest of the team which, if the team chemistry is right, can be fun. When film processing facilities are available the evenings can also mean checking through film, so sleep becomes low on the list of the stylist's priorities. To bed after midnight with another 5am start is the schedule that must be kept up for days at a time.

Once back from the trip, the film editing process begins, which, like advertising, may or may not require input from the stylist. At the same time, meetings with clients are being scheduled to plan the next trip.

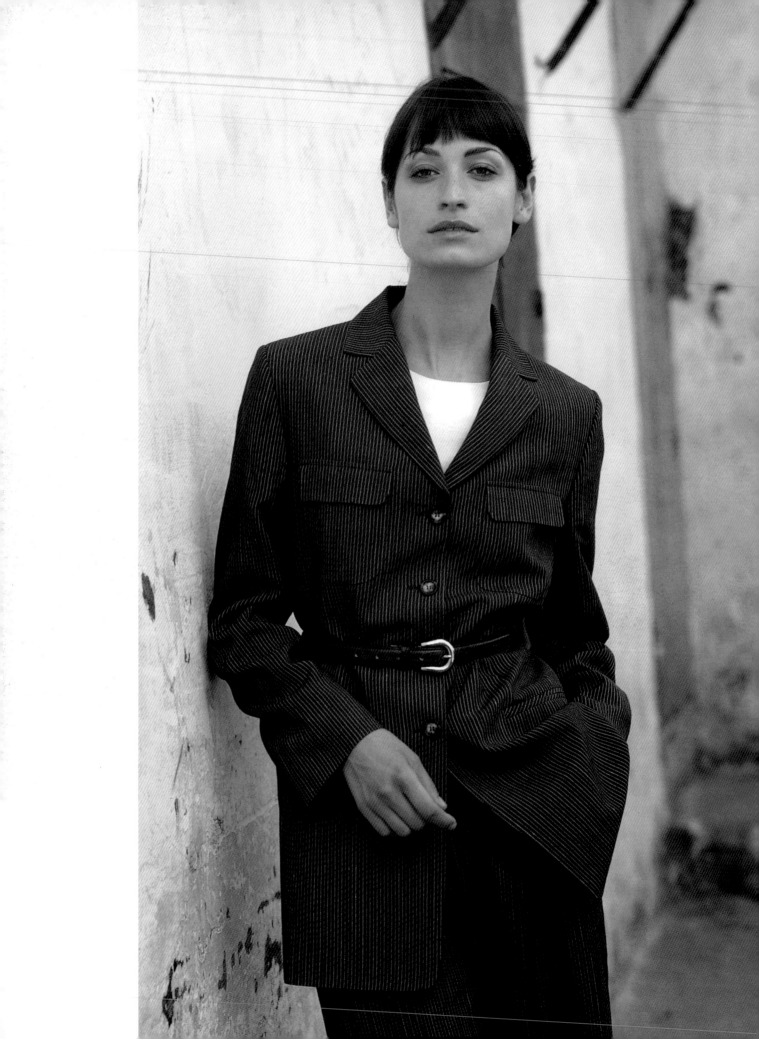

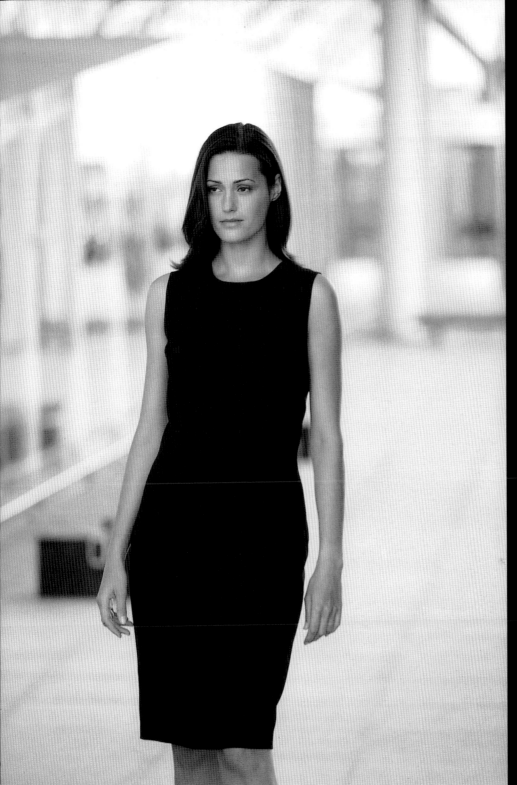

Photographer: Steffano Massimo for Next Directory

Photographer: Eamon McCabe for Next Directory

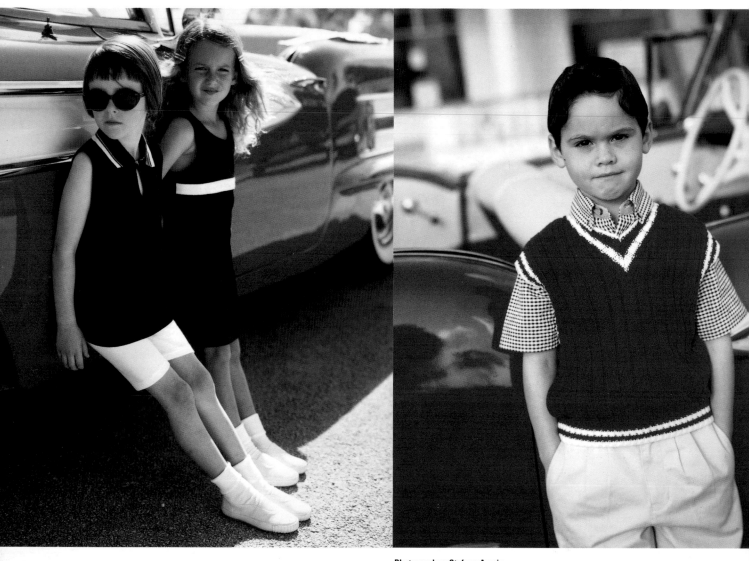

Photographer: Stefano Azario

Stylist: Helen Crowther

Art Direction: Davies Baron for Mothercare UK Ltd

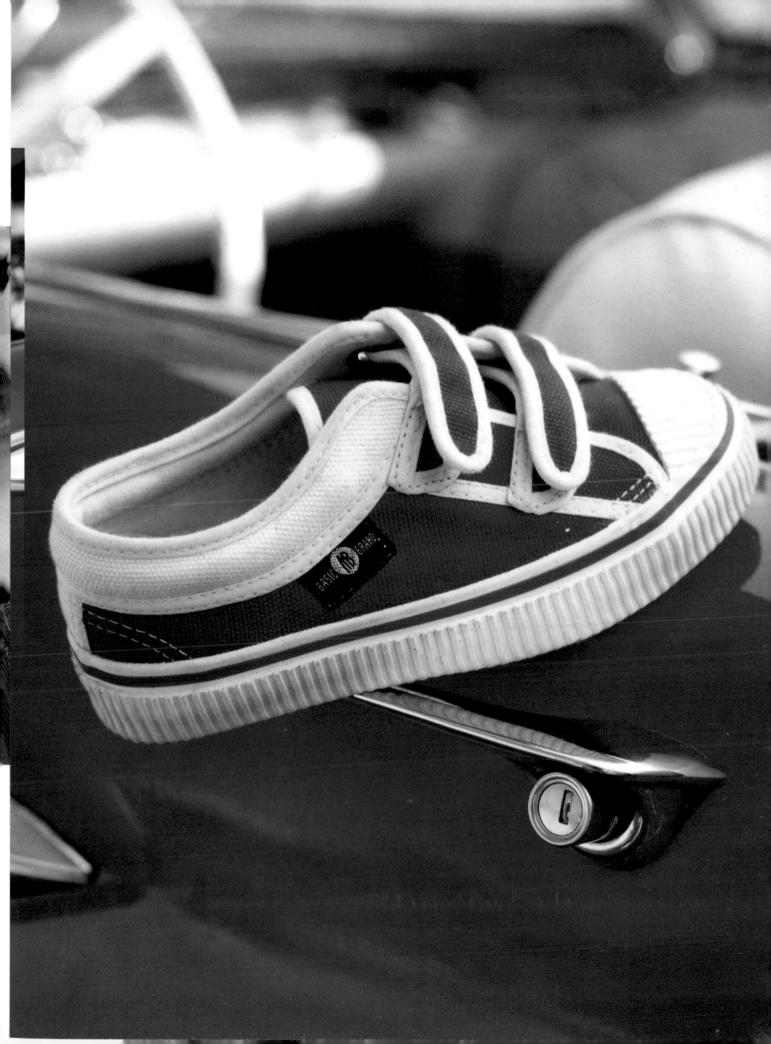

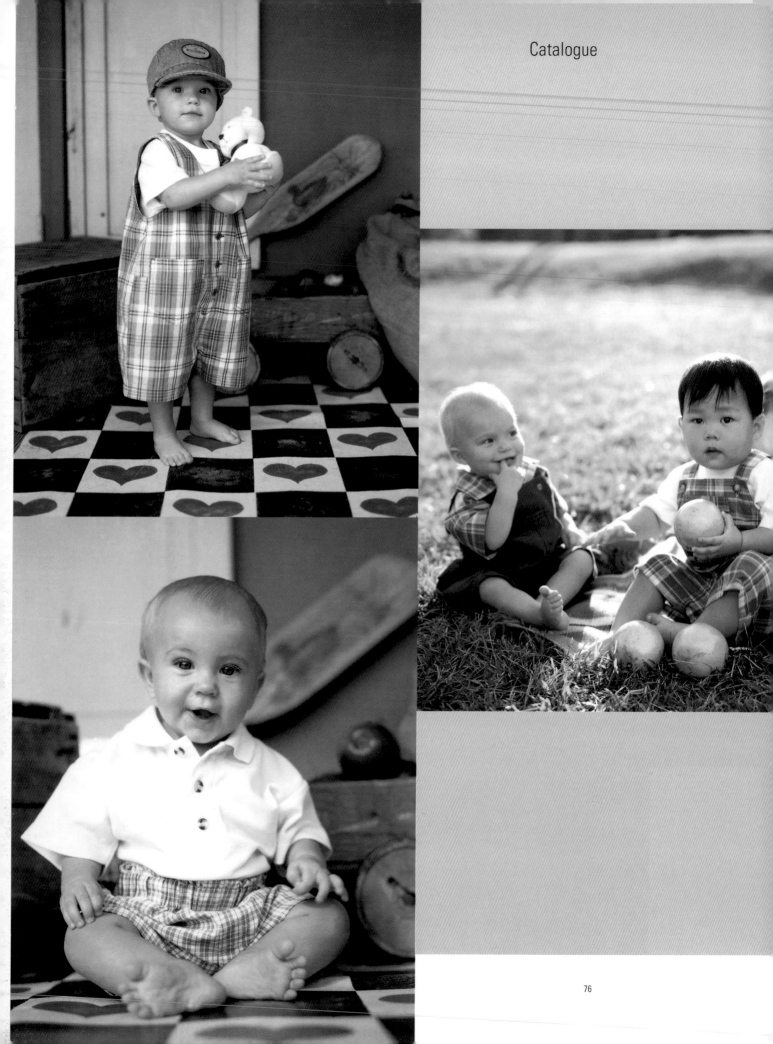

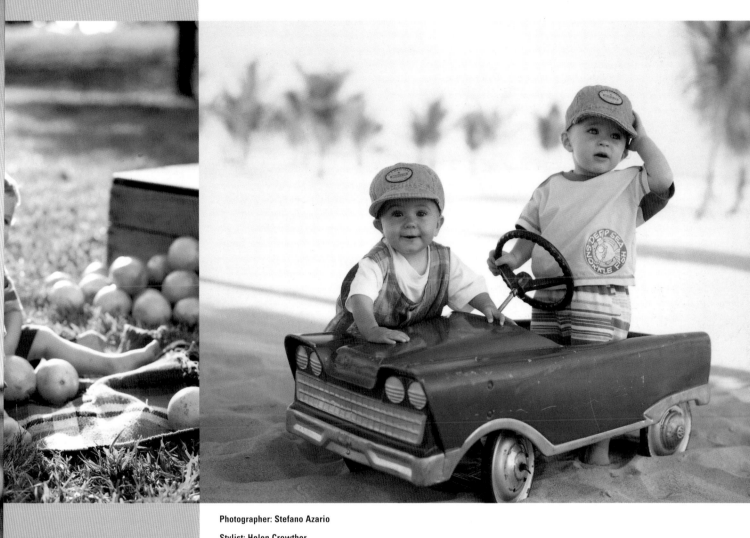

Photographer: Stefano Azario

Stylist: Helen Crowther

Art Direction: Davies Baron for Mothercare UK Ltd

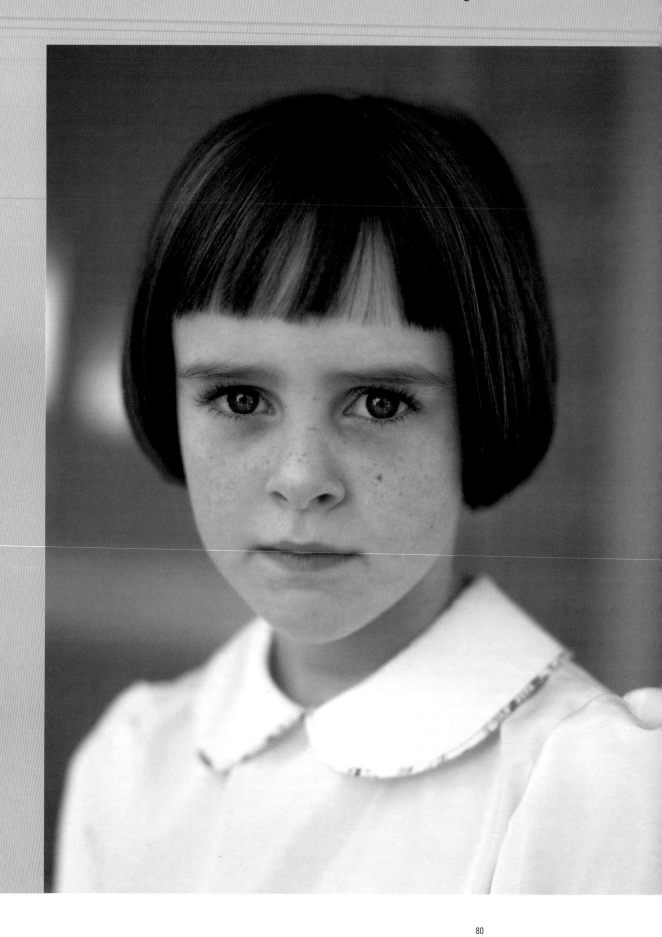

Photographer: Stefano Azario

Stylist: Helen Crowther

Art Direction: Davies Baron for Mothercare UK Ltd

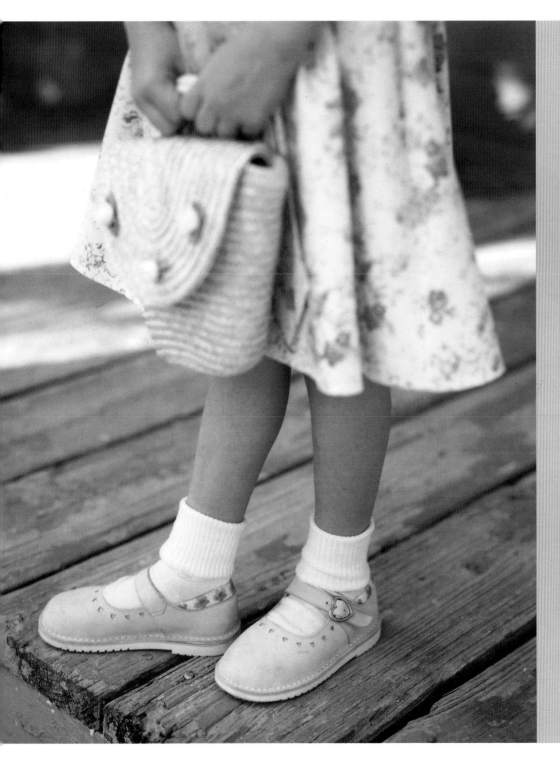

Music promo

Music promos are very much a vehicle for the artist(s). The promo theme and styling may take inspiration from an idea that has nothing to do with what is deemed fashionable and is furthest removed from the season's fashion stories. However, sometimes an injection of fashion direction is what is called for. The original idea for the promo is usually the combined effort of the video director, record company and the artist(s). Because of the huge scale of many music promos - lavish sets, lighting techniques and computer-generated images - the stylist's input is, more often than not, the icing on the cake. This does not mean that it is an easier task than any other area of styling. Music promo shoots are notorious for their gruelling schedules - 6am call times and 4am wrap times - and their unfriendly locations where the logistics of dressing artists and extras makes it all the harder. This is not work for the faint hearted and, because music promos often involve many extras (dancers, backing singers and other performers), the video stylist needs access to reliable and quick witted assistants. Music promos can open up extraordinary styling possibilities and this can be enormously exciting and creative. It is one of the few areas where styling begins to overlap with costume design and the video stylist is no stranger to the sewing machine. If the video director wants something specific, then it must be found, and if it cannot be found, it will often need to be made. Rather than a portfolio, the video stylist keeps a showreel - short edited excerpts of past promos - which is sent out by the agent to directors, production companies and record companies.

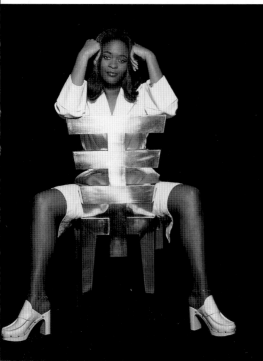

Artist: Beverlei Brown, SideStep/Network Records
Photographer: Neil McKenzie Matthews
Art Direction: Blue Evolution

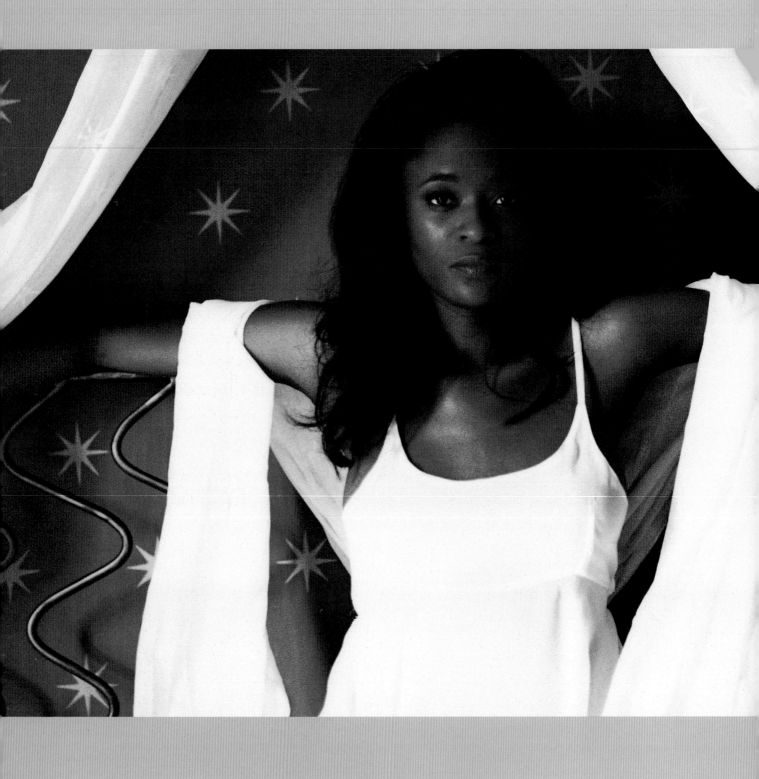

Music promo starts with a meeting involving the record company or the production company and the video director. It is at this meeting that the stylist sees the storyboard - a detailed drawing of each shot - and listens to the music to get a feel for the band/artist and the promo. Usually, the director has a very clear idea of what is required and will explain which parts of the promo need specific outfits and which require original ideas from the stylist. Ideas are discussed there and then, with little time to think. Some promos need something a little more theatrical and may require costume changes throughout to illustrate different parts of the story.

In theory, the stylist will get to meet the band prior to the shoot. This will make clear the direction the band wants to project. Taking the band shopping with the advance budget is often the best way to achieve the results required. In practice, bands with busy gig and recording schedules are notoriously difficult to meet, or even to communicate with, therefore the video stylist takes on enormous responsibility when choosing outfits and must thoroughly question the record company about the changing likes and dislikes of the band and research past images in order to get the look right.

The stylist must be careful to assess whether or not the budget is realistic at the first meeting and to speak up if it is not. Keeping within the budget, the stylist buys, hires and makes - or has made - outfits that fit the brief. Prior to hiring or buying, it makes sense to Polaroid garments and show them to the director, along with visual references of outfits to be made. If the budget is tight, extras are often asked to bring certain clothes with them and, with a solo artist, the stylist often works with the artist's own wardrobe of clothes and accessories and adds to it.

Styling new bands from scratch has great possibilities for creative work. When promoting a new artist the look is make-or-break, with huge financial sums riding on the success of the launch.

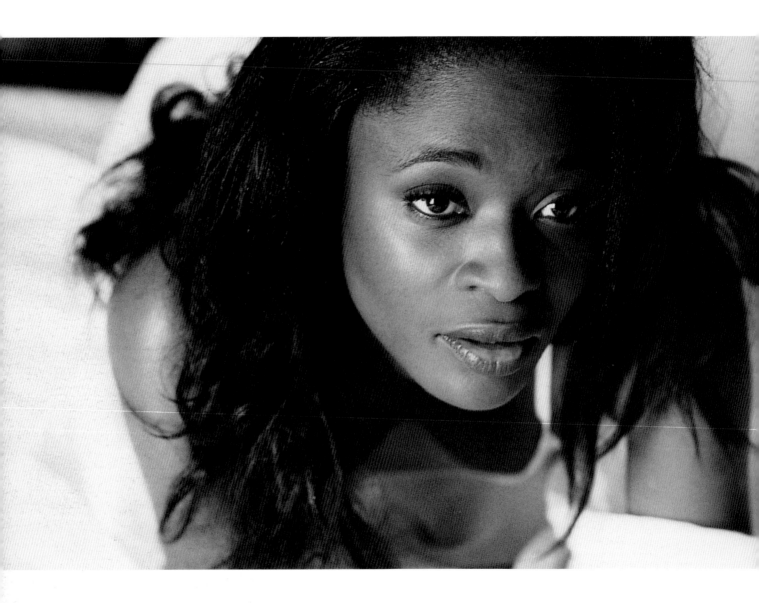

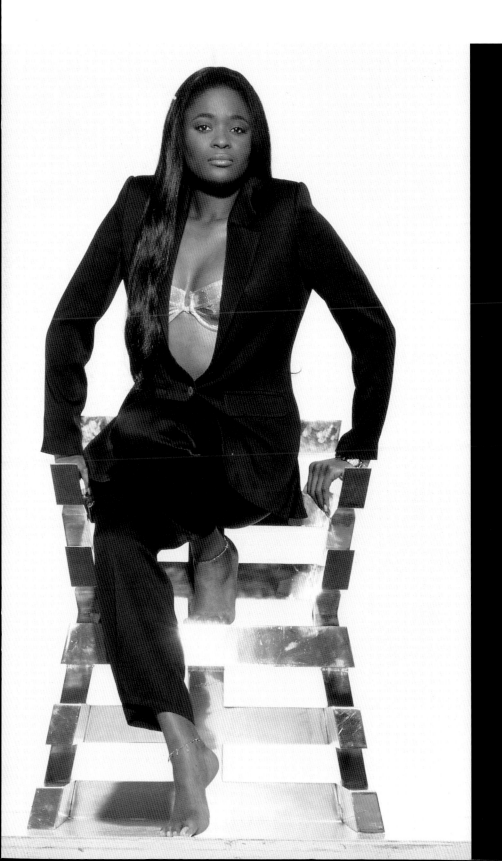

Hair and make-up is an integral part of the image on a music promo. In order to communicate successfully with the target audience, the complete image must be spot on. The stylist and director brief the hair and make-up team and explain the clothes and storyboard to them. It is important to do this prior to the shoot as their ideas may require testing or preparation and they may need time.

At the shoot, time is the important factor and the stylist, hair stylist and make-up artist should be punctual and have prepared and at hand everything they need for each shot on the storyboard. If the director is available, it is a good idea for the stylist to try all the outfits on the artists for final approval. It may be necessary for the director to do a quick lighting test with the most important outfits. If there is a problem with the way they look on set, it will be the clothes that need to be changed not the lighting, and the stylist will be expected to have suitable alternatives. The stylist, hair stylist and make-up artist should have finished preparing the band or artist by the time they are called for the first shot. On set, it is important to watch the monitor (the screen that shows what is being filmed) during filming and be on hand with kit bags to do touch ups and make adjustments where necessary. As each scene is shot, it is ticked off the storyboard. The stylist should check with the director that the scene is definitely finished (shooting on film, the first assistant director needs to check the gate and on video, they often need to see the play back). When the all clear is given, the outfits and hair and make-up are changed for the next scene and the process repeated until the director calls a wrap.

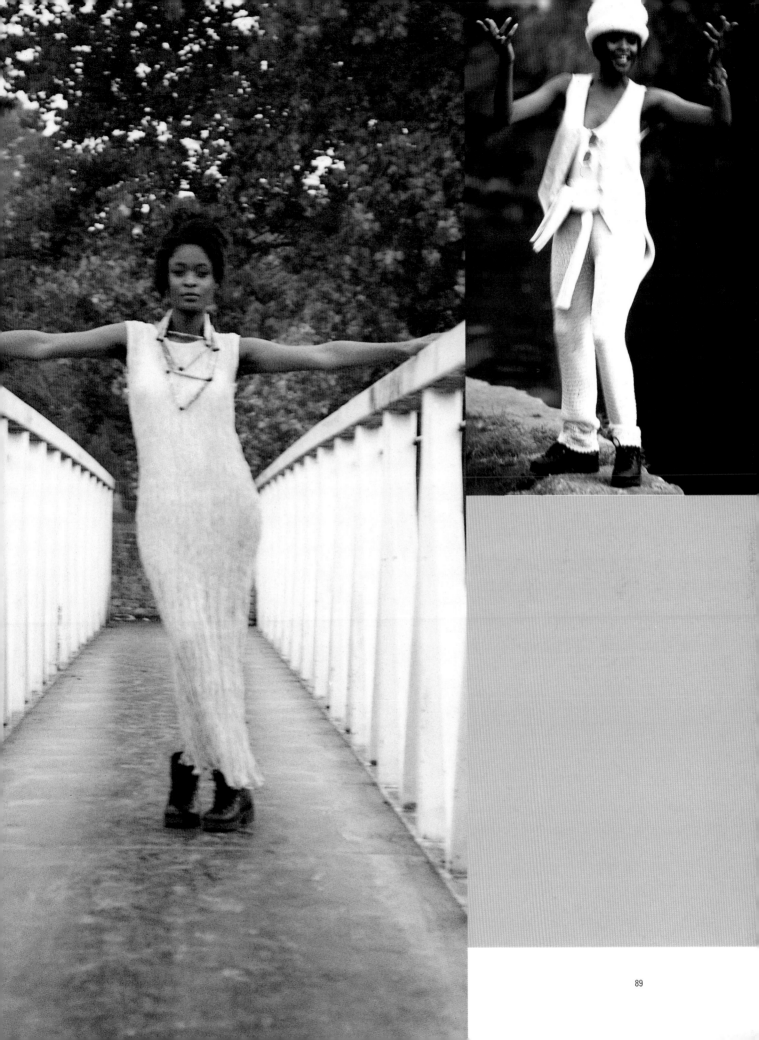

The future

The role of the stylist, like that of many other professions within the fashion industry, is changing and expanding. As it overlaps with that of the art director, many stylists are taking on board more overall responsibility for the finished image, making a greater contribution to fashion images as a whole. Stylists are being employed as consultants in many areas. When working for designers, they not only direct the way that clothes are styled but also contribute ideas for fabrics, colours and shapes at the drawing board - the starting point of a clothing collection. Stylists are in demand from public figures for image consultancy and from major fashion companies for product launches. It can be a rewarding and satisfying career both creatively and financially.

For hair stylists and make-up artists the future lies in product development. Many hair stylists are launching their own brand of hair products and make-up artists are consultants on ranges for big cosmetic houses or are launching their own brands of make-up.

Trunk shows, where designers sell direct to the public from the runway, are an employment growth area for stylists, hair stylists and make-up artists.

New technology, like CD-ROM, fashion on the internet and on-line publishing, mean that the areas are growing within which fashion's image-makers can find work.

The styling kit

As explained in the preceding sections, the stylist's
role differs according to the nature of each individual
project brief. However the tools of the trade remain pretty
much the same. It is important that kits are kept updated
and tidy so that on the shoot or show day the stylist is fully
prepared for every eventuality and no time is wasted.

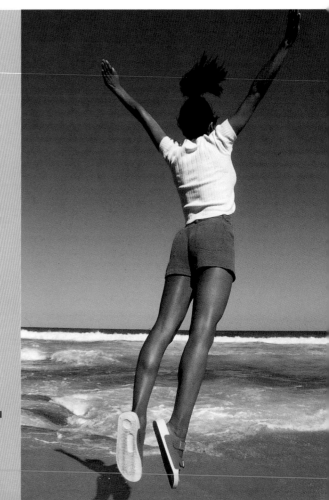

Photograph © Heather Flavell

Iron and ironing board or a steamer
Probably the most important pieces of equipment. On some jobs it is better to have both as an iron is good to provide crispness, as for classic cotton shirts, whilst a steamer is the easiest and quickest way to smooth tailoring. On show days, these are handed over to the dressers who are in charge of pressing all the garments.

Bull dog clips Usually for photographic stills, these are used for clipping in clothes at the back to give an outfit a narrower, more streamlined shape. Especially useful if clothes are too big at the waistline.

Toupee tape Available from hairdressing supplies stores, this double-sided tape is handy because, unlike most adhesive tapes, it adheres to skin. If clothes are not sitting where they should, they can simply be taped on. It is also useful for turning up hems on skirts and trousers when there is no time to sew.

Nail scissors The fine point on these scissors makes them ideal for trimming the tiny loose threads which invariably show up on stills pictures. Also, if garments are too small, it is sometimes possible to unpick seams for a better fit without damaging the garment.

Gaffer tape This strong adhesive tape can be used instead of bull dog clips on the back of garments to narrow and pinch garments in areas where bull dog clips may be hard to conceal.

Marker pens Black marker pens can be used to colour in black shoes where samples are worn and faded. Especially good on black suede.

Blu-tac Used to get marks off clothes, especially pen or pencil off leather. Also good for repositioning drooping buttons. When buttons are catching the light on stills pictures, a small wedge of blu-tac underneath will fix it at the angle that is best for the light.

Safety pins For pinning clothes in if they are too big, especially trouser or skirt waists. Also for pinning up trouser hems.

Pins, needles and threads Stylists are expected to do a lot of sewing and repairing. This could be anything from hemming to re-sewing buttons to quite major alterations.

Parcel tape During runway shows and stills photography, this wide brown tape can be wrapped around the hand, sticky side out, to dust down clothes. It is especially effective on dark or pale coloured clothes.

Masking tape An alternative for dusting clothes; also used in strips to mask the soles of shoes that are slipping on the runway.

Inner soles Invariably, the shoes for a shoot or runway show will not fit the models. Inner soles can be cut to size or used in layers to make big shoes fit.

First aid kit Especially useful on location shoots and abroad where first aid facilities may not be available.

Insect spray Again, especially for locations or trips abroad.

Spare underwear A smooth flesh-toned underwired bra and a g-string are always useful as underwear may show through certain clothes.

Tippex Can be useful to touch out small marks on white clothes.

Scissors A must for many purposes, from cutting tape to trimming inner soles to scoring the soles of new shoes to stop them slipping on the runway.

Shoulder pads or wadding To achieve a perfect fit, especially with tailoring, these are a must.

Index